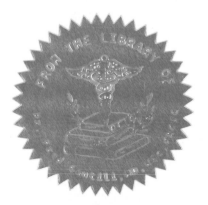

CLINICAL APPLICATION OF BLOOD GASES

CLINICAL APPLICATION OF
BLOOD GASES

Second Edition

Barry A. Shapiro, M.D.
Associate Professor of Clinical Anesthesia and Physical
Medicine, Northwestern University Medical School;
Medical Director, Department of Respiratory Therapy,
Northwestern Memorial Hospital

Ronald A. Harrison, M.D.
Assistant Professor of Clinical Anesthesia, Northwestern
University Medical School;
Associate Medical Director, Department of Respiratory
Therapy, Northwestern Memorial Hospital

John R. Walton, B.S., A.R.R.T.
Director, Department of Respiratory Therapy, Northwestern
Memorial Hospital

YEAR BOOK MEDICAL PUBLISHERS, INC.
CHICAGO • LONDON

Reprinted, October 1973
Reprinted, February 1974
Reprinted, January 1975
Reprinted, March 1976
Second Edition, May 1977

Library of Congress Catalog Card Number: 76-53233

International Standard Book Number: 0-8151-7638-4

To David, Leslie, Nancy and Erika

Foreword to the Second Edition

THE RAPID PROGRESS of critical-care medicine and cardiopulmonary supportive technology in the past five years calls for update and expansion of CLINICAL APPLICATION OF BLOOD GASES. The general approach and some of the concepts put forth in the first edition were considered controversial and in many cases not well documented. However, over the past five years, a large majority of these concepts have become accepted and well documented in the medical literature. In addition, the idea that respiratory acid-base imbalance should be considered a *primary* ventilatory phenomenon is far less controversial today than five years ago. I owe a great deal to the supporters and critics of the first edition, for they have provided the basis for this revision.

Although the general approach of the text remains unchanged, the scope and depth of the material have been significantly expanded. To accomplish this, I am privileged to be joined in authorship by Ronald Harrison and John Walton. Doctor Harrison possesses a wealth of knowledge in cardiopulmonary physiology and its clinical application; Mr. Walton has knowledge and experience in blood gas technology and its application that are second to none. The improvements and expansions in this revision are due primarily to their efforts.

BARRY A. SHAPIRO, M.D.

Preface to the Second Edition

IT IS HOPED that this book will provide for respiratory therapists and critical-care nurses a basic text for understanding the clinical application of blood gas measurements. In addition, selective reading should provide a valuable resource and a clinical introduction for medical students and physicians. To accomplish this diversity, we have divided the text into four sections. Section I consists of four chapters dealing with the basic chemistry and physics upon which respiratory and acid-base physiology is based. These chapters are presented at a basic level and may be omitted by the more sophisticated reader. The second section is comprised of seven chapters dealing with the physiology of respiration and acid-base balance that is germane to blood gas interpretation. The third section contains three chapters that discuss the guidelines and methods recommended for proper clinical interpretation of blood gas measurements. Section IV contains the basic clinical information necessary for properly applying blood gas measurements to the critically ill patient.

Our intent is not to provide a complete text of respiratory physiology, acid-base physiology, and acute medicine. Rather, we strive to provide the basic information necessary to properly apply blood gas measurements in the care of the critically ill and to present the material in a form as readable and comprehensible as possible without excessive oversimplification. Frequent referencing to current literature is provided primarily for those interested in further reading or those who wish to review the original publications upon which concepts and guidelines are based.

ACKNOWLEDGMENTS

We wish to thank our colleagues, Dr. Edward Brunner, Dr. James Eckenhoff, Dr. John Ditzler, Dr. Ralph Braunschweig, Dr. Richard Davison, and Dr. John Buehler for their invaluable criticisms, suggestions, and support.

The aid and assistance of our colleagues in Respiratory Therapy at Northwestern Memorial Hospital are appreciated, especially Robert Kacmarek, A.R.R.T.; John Peterson, A.R.R.T.; Carole Trout, R.N., A.R.R.T.; Elizabeth Vostinak, R.N., A.R.R.T.; Camille Woodward, R.N., A.R.R.T.; and the entire supervisory staff.

The development and maintenance of an accurate, efficient, and progressive Northwestern Memorial Hospital Central Blood Gas Laboratory have been due in great measure to our supervisor, Michael Steiner, A.R.R.T., and his associates.

The imagination and technical excellence of the medical illustrations are entirely due to the talents of Jennifer Giancarlo. The manuscript was developed and prepared by Patti Hara, who has our special thanks for her patience, loyalty, and superb performance.

B. SHAPIRO
R. HARRISON
J. WALTON

Foreword to the First Edition

IN THE EARLY 1950s many clinicians assumed that an arbitrary "normal" blood pressure was necessary to sustain life. With little concern for maintaining blood flow to vital organs, an attempt was usually made to keep systolic blood pressure, measured by indirect and imprecise methods, above 100 mm Hg. As a result, for a decade few patients died in shock or from an acute illness without having received an infusion of the pressor substance norepinephrine, sometimes in extraordinary concentration. At autopsy, pathologic evidence of excessive vasoconstriction was often apparent, raising questions as to whether the disease or the treatment was responsible for death. Today, this practice has waned and less attention is paid to an arbitrary blood pressure level; more thought is given to the basic principles of cardiovascular regulation, vasopressors are used less frequently, more fluid is given to expand the vascular space, and therapy is directed at specific components of the cardiovascular system.

We appear to be in the middle of another, similar cycle, also concerning clinical physiologic measurements, namely, blood gas determinations. These values, like blood pressure, are subject to errors in measurement as well as errors in sampling and handling. As with blood pressure, blood gases are valid only at the instant the measurement is made and do not reveal anything about the status of tissue perfusion.

The periodic measurement of blood gases in sick patients was not common until the mid-1960s. Even today, the analyses are usually not available in small hospitals, and in many teaching hospitals blood gases can be obtained readily only from 8 A.M. to 5 P.M. These determinations have been accorded great importance in diagnosis and monitoring patient care, especially in acute medicine—so much so that there are those who appear to believe that if blood gases were measured, then the patient obviously had received the best possible care. If the findings were within normal limits and the patient died, nothing more could have been done; if the results were abnormal and the patient died, then the cause of death was apparent.

Measurement of blood oxygen or carbon dioxide tension and hydrogen ion concentration yields information otherwise unobtainable, but such analyses cannot be considered independently of other laboratory tests or clinical observations any more than can a high specific gravity of urine, a low hematocrit or a high body temperature. This is only one of a series of tests and it must be placed in perspective. Doctor Shapiro proposes to do this in his monograph — and I think he does it well!

JAMES E. ECKENHOFF, M.D.

Professor of Anesthesia and Dean,
Northwestern University Medical School

Preface to the First Edition

MEDICAL THERAPY is based upon the diagnosis of disease and the application of medications and techniques to reverse or control the disease process. The last three decades have witnessed an expansion of medicine to include diagnostic and therapeutic techniques that are impressively complex and sophisticated. Today's medicine and surgery can cure many diseases if the patient can be kept alive and physiologically intact while the cure is being effected. Such diagnostic and therapeutic advances have demanded that more time and effort be devoted to supporting the vital systems.

Acute supportive medicine — critical-care medicine — demands the same discipline and scientific approach that have already been established in diagnostic and therapeutic medical and paramedical areas. This supportive approach is quite familiar to the medical discipline of anesthesiology. To accomplish complex and sophisticated surgical procedures it is necessary to support the vital systems while rendering the patient insensible to pain. An example of the increasing sophistication of acute supportive medicine is the anesthesiologist's application of his techniques and methodology to respiratory care. Similarly, the single most important technical advance of the past decade in cardiopulmonary supportive medicine has been the clinical availability of arterial blood gas measurement. The anesthesiologist's clinical application of these laboratory measurements has had great impact on the field of respiratory care.

The traditional approach to blood gas interpretation is totally in terms of acid-base balance. Respiratory acidosis and alkalosis are universal terms, even though these acid-base imbalances are the result of primary ventilatory changes. This indirect terminology makes clinical application of blood gas measurements confusing. Most patients in whom blood gas analysis is indicated do not have primary metabolic acid-base disturbance; rather, the great majority have cardiopulmonary disease.

There would be no need to redefine the traditional concepts and to introduce new terminology if these concepts were readily applied to the clinical supportive care of cardiopulmonary disease. However, anyone teaching or learning the clinical applications of blood gas measurement in the critically ill patient recognizes that a clinically practical approach is very much needed — an approach in which the primary interpretation would reflect the primary physiologic abnormality requiring supportive therapy. The approach put forth in this book has been developed from clinical experience in supportive medicine and is based on the clinical application of blood gases to the critically ill patient. If any defense for changing the system is necessary, it is based solely on the fact that these changes make blood gas measurements readily applicable to the supportive therapy of critically ill patients. This makes blood gas analysis clinically meaningful and appropriate in critical-care medicine.

It is hoped this book will provide a basic text for the respiratory therapist and the critical-care nurse, a clinical introduction and physiologic review for the medical student, and a practical approach to cardiopulmonary supportive medicine for the accomplished physician. Part I is devoted to basic respiratory physiology, Part II to the clinical *interpretation* of arterial blood gases, and Part III to the clinical *application* of arterial blood gases. To make the text as readable and comprehensible as possible, technical information, exercises, and case studies have been placed in the appendix. Because complete referencing within the text would make it tedious and clumsy, a list (Selected References) is provided in a separate section. A glossary is appended for those who may be unfamiliar with basic scientific and clinical nomenclature.

The reader will find that the clinical confusion surrounding blood gases no longer exists if the physiology in Part I is understood and if the concepts and terminology in Parts II and III are accepted. Proper application of blood gas measurements to the supportive care of critically ill patients is essential. To that end this book is dedicated.

BARRY A. SHAPIRO, M.D.

Table of Contents

The Basic Chemistry and Physics Related to Blood Gas Analysis

EXPERIENCE HAS SHOWN that much of the confusion surrounding blood gas and acid-base interpretation results from inadequate comprehension of basic physics and chemistry. These first four chapters are designed as an introduction for the novice and as reference chapters for the initiated. They assume that the reader has no previous knowledge of the material; however, even for the more sophisticated reader the review should prove beneficial.

1 / The Physics of Gases

THE EXCHANGE of gas molecules across permeable membranes (respiration) is a physical phenomenon essential to the maintenance of life. Like all molecules, gas molecules are constantly in motion and are randomly colliding with each other and with various surfaces. The nature of these gas molecules dictates three intuitive truths:

1. The gas occupies a volume. The nature of that volume and the number of gas molecules affect the behavior of the gas.

2. The gas exerts a pressure within the volume. The frequency of the random collisions of the molecules against the sides of the container determines the pressure.

3. The gas has a temperature because molecular movement is a process of heat expenditure. This temperature determines how fast the molecules move.

Intuitive understanding may be a helpful beginning, but we must fully comprehend the physics and chemistry involved before extending these generalities to the clinical setting.

Matter is defined as the material from which physical substances are formed. Matter exists in three primary forms on the earth's surface: solid, liquid, and gas. Gases are distinguished from other states of matter by their ability to expand without limit to fill the available space and to exert pressure uniformly on all surfaces. Knowledge of certain physical properties of gases (e.g., volume, temperature, pressure) is essential for understanding their behavior.

1. *Volume* refers to the space that a gas occupies and is measured in terms of cubic centimeters (cc) or milliliters (ml).

2. *Pressure* is defined mathematically as force per unit area. In practice, the measurement is obtained by noting the height to which the force can support a column of mercury. This is most often expressed as millimeters of mercury (mm Hg).*

On the earth's surface, gas molecules are in constant motion (kinetic movement). Such molecular movement produces heat. Quantitation of the heat is called *temperature.*

3. *Temperature* is classically measured with a thermometer—an instrument that registers a change in volume in response to a change in heat. Volume changes due to heat variability are carefully calibrat-

---

*The classic mercury scale is known as the *Torricelli scale;* often the units of the Torricelli scale (mm Hg) are referred to as *Torr.*

ed at reproducible points in various liquids, e.g., the boiling point and freezing point of water. Using standard substances such as mercury or alcohol, these incremental changes in volume are measured and so-called temperature scales are derived. There are three temperature scales commonly used today—the Fahrenheit, centigrade, and Kelvin scales.

The Fahrenheit scale is seldom used in medicine although it is the most commonly used temperature scale in the United States. On this scale the freezing point of water is set at 32 degrees and the boiling point of water at 212 degrees.

The centigrade (Celsius) scale is so designed that the total change in volume from the freezing point of water (zero degrees) to the boiling point of water (100 degrees) is divided into 100 equal increments. This is the most common temperature scale used in medicine and is considered the metric temperature scale.

The Kelvin (absolute) temperature scale utilizes the same incremental volume changes per degree as does the centigrade scale. However, zero degrees Kelvin is equal to −273 degrees centigrade—a temperature that theoretically represents the point where all molecular movement ceases; this is called absolute zero.

When comparing the behavior of different gases (or different amounts of the same gas) it is necessary to quantitate the amount of gas (i.e., the number of molecules) present in the sample. Although gas particles are small, they do have a mass. When mass is measured in relation to the earth's gravitational force it is called *weight*. The mass or weight of a defined amount of gas is quantitated by *Avogadro's number;* that is, 6.023×10^{23} molecules of any gas will equal one gram molecular weight (gram atomic weight).

When referring to gases in physical chemistry, n stands for the number of molecules in a gas sample.* This allows for the comparison of different gases by knowing both their atomic weight and the weight of the respective sample.

The Gas Laws

From physical chemistry it is known that all gases behave in an "ideally" predictable fashion at exceedingly low pressures—commonly referred to as the behavior of an "ideal gas." Real gases behave in extremely complicated ways at great extremes of pressure; how-

---

*When $n = 1$, it means that the measured weight of that gaseous substance in grams is numerically equal to its gram atomic weight.

ever, in the range of pressures found at the earth's surface the behavior of these real gases closely approximates that of the ideal gas. A mathematical relationship known as the *ideal gas law* has been developed to describe the behavior of these real gases under conditions found at the earth's surface:

$$P \times V = nR \times T$$

P is pressure in atmospheres — one atmosphere equals 760 mm Hg; V is volume in liters (L) — one milliliter (ml) equals one thousandth of a liter; T is temperature on the Kelvin scale; n equals the amount of gas present; and R is the gas constant — a fixed value of 0.082 which is expressed in liter atmospheres per mole degree. Mathematically, R is referred to as a constant of proportionality and allows for the interrelationship of the various properties of the gas, such as pressure, volume, and temperature.

Using the ideal gas law, if the amount of gas remains constant (i.e., n remains constant) the interrelationships of temperature, pressure, and volume under differing sets of conditions may be predicted. In other words, assuming nR is constant:

$$\frac{P_1 \times V_1}{T_1} = \frac{P_2 \times V_2}{T_2}$$

Note that if one of the three terms (P, V, T) remains unchanged while another changes its value, the third term must change in a predictable manner. When any one value remains unchanged, the three possible relationships are as follows:

1. Boyle's law: $P_1 \times V_1 = P_2 \times V_2$

Boyle's law states that if temperature remains constant, pressure will vary inversely with volume. The disease tuberculosis (TB) is a useful mnemonic: T = Temperature constant, B = Boyle's law.

2. Charles' law: $\dfrac{V_1}{T_1} = \dfrac{V_2}{T_2}$

Charles' law states that if pressure is held constant, volume and temperature will vary directly. The disease cerebral palsy (CP) is a useful mnemonic: C = Charles' law; P = pressure constant.

3. Gay-Lussac's law: $\dfrac{P_1}{T_1} = \dfrac{P_2}{T_2}$

Gay-Lussac's law states that if volume is held constant, pressure and temperature will vary directly. Vitamin G is a useful mnemonic: V = volume constant; G = Gay-Lussac's law.

Partial Pressure of Gases

The earth's atmosphere is composed primarily of gas molecules. These molecules have mass and are attracted toward the earth's center by the force of gravity. At the earth's surface this atmospheric weight exerts a pressure sufficient to support a column of mercury 760 mm high. This *atmospheric pressure* affects everything on the earth's surface; life forms are no exception.

The earth's atmosphere is composed of varying amounts of several different gases, therefore understanding the behavior of gases when they are mixed together is imperative. *Dalton's law* summarizes a very important physical principle pertaining to the mixture of gases: *In a mixture of gases the total pressure is equal to the sum of the partial pressures of the separate components* (Fig 1–1). It is sometimes easier to think of a partial pressure of a component gas as the pressure that gas would exert if it were present alone in the system. In other words, since each of the individual gases may be considered as acting independently, its contribution to the total pressure is dependent upon what fraction or percent of the total gases it occupies (Table 1–1).[14]

Fig 1–1.—A simplified illustration of the principle of partial pressures according to Dalton's law. The three *squares* represent containers of equal volumes and constant temperatures. The *circles* represent gas molecules in motion. The pressure within the container is the result of gas molecules colliding with the sides of the container.

If four molecules of gas A *(black circles)* are present, the total pressure may be theoretically expressed as 4; if five molecules of gas B *(white circles)* are present, the total pressure may be theoretically expressed as 5; if a mixture of gases A and B is present, the total pressure may be theoretically expressed as 9.

Since the total pressure of 9 is the sum of the partial pressures (i.e., partial pressure of gas A is 4, partial pressure of gas B is 5), the pressure exerted by each individual gas is the same whether it occupies the space by itself or is present in a mixture of other gases.

PRESSURE = 4   PRESSURE = 5   PRESSURE = 9

  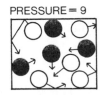

TABLE 1-1.—PARTIAL PRESSURES OF COMPONENT
GASES COMPRISING AIR UNDER VARIOUS CONDITIONS

COMPONENT GAS	PERCENT OF TOTAL GAS	PARTIAL PRESSURE (mm Hg)
Air at sea level (760 mm Hg)		
Oxygen (O_2)	20.9	159
Nitrogen (N_2)	79.0	600
Others	0.1	1
Ideal *alveolar gas* at sea level (760 mm Hg) (air sample)		
Oxygen (O_2)	13.3	101
Nitrogen (N_2)	75.2	572
Carbon dioxide (CO_2)	5.3	40
Water vapor (H_2O)	6.2	47
Air at 18,000 ft above sea level (380 mm Hg)		
Oxygen (O_2)	20.9	79.4
Nitrogen (N_2)	79.0	300.2
Others	0.1	0.4
Ideal *alveolar gas* at 18,000 ft above sea level (380 mm Hg) (air sample)		
Oxygen (O_2)	5.9	22
Nitrogen (N_2)	73.9	271
Carbon dioxide (CO_2)	10.6	40
Water vapor (H_2O)	12.4	47

It is worth reemphasizing that the partial pressure of a gas is dependent upon the number of molecules existing in that fixed space; the pressure that gas exerts is unaffected by changes of other gas molecules. For example, physical laws render it improper to say that the partial pressure of oxygen decreases because the partial pressure of carbon dioxide increases. Remember, each gas acts independently—as if it alone occupied the space.

Water Vapor Pressure

Some substances exist in more than one state of matter under certain environmental conditions. Within a given range of temperatures and pressures, water can exist as a liquid, a gas, or a solid.* Water in the gaseous form is called *water vapor* or molecular water and is re-

---

*When a substance such as H_2O exists simultaneously in both the liquid and gaseous phases, the partial pressure it exerts as a gas is directly related to the existing temperature. In general the partial pressure of the gas increases as the temperature increases until it equals the ambient pressure, at which point the liquid (H_2O) boils.

ferred to as *humidity*. When water vapor exists in a mixture of gases it follows the gas laws and exerts a partial pressure.[10]

Alveolar gas is 100% humidified at body temperature, therefore "ideal" alveolar gas contains a water vapor pressure (PH_2O) of 47 mm Hg. Remember, water vapor is a gas and follows all the physical principles applicable to other gases.[7]

BTPS

Clinical measurements are usually accomplished under "standard" conditions. In blood gas measurement the standard conditions are body temperature and pressure fully saturated (BTPS).[7] Body temperature is 37°C; the pressure is the atmospheric pressure to which the body is exposed; saturated refers to maximum water vapor at 37°C, which is 47 mm Hg.

Diffusion and Blood Gas Solubility

The constant random movement of gas molecules results in the movement of those molecules from an area of relatively high concentration toward an area of lower concentration. This net passive movement of gas molecules is called *diffusion*.* All life is dependent upon the ability of gas molecules to cross cell membranes. This process of *gas diffusion* across a semipermeable membrane occurs primarily in response to a pressure gradient; that is, the pressure on one side of the membrane must be greater than the pressure on the other side. In general, the greater the pressure difference, the faster will be the net movement of molecules. *Each gas moves according to its own pressure gradient without regard to what other gases in the mixture may be doing.* Net movement stops when the partial pressures are equal on both sides, a situation referred to as a state of *dynamic equilibrium*.[14]

If a membrane separates a gas mixture from a liquid, the degree to which the gases can dissolve in the liquid will affect the diffusion process. In general, when a gas is exposed to a liquid, the gas molecules move into the liquid and become dissolved unless they combine chemically with constituents of the liquid. Eventually the number of gas molecules leaving the liquid equals the number of gas molecules entering the liquid, and a state of dynamic equilibrium is established.[10] In other words, the pressure of the gases in the liquid will

---

*The presence of a semipermeable membrane, such as the alveolar capillary membrane of the lung, can be visualized as a limiting factor allowing for only selective diffusion of certain substances.

then be equal to the pressure of the gases in the atmosphere or, more exactly, the *partial pressures in solution* will be equal to the atmospheric partial pressures. *Henry's law* states that the amount of gas that can be dissolved in a liquid is proportional to the partial pressure of the gas to which the liquid is exposed.[7]

Thus, we can see that the diffusion process across the alveolar capillary membrane will be primarily dependent upon the partial pressure gradients across the membrane. There are several other factors that determine how effectively gas will diffuse across the alveolar capillary membrane. One factor is the weight of the gas and is expressed in *Graham's law*. This law states that the diffusibility of a gas is inversely proportional to the square root of its molecular weight; in other words, the heavier the molecule, the less its diffusibility.[14]

2 / Chemistry of Acid-Base Balance

AN ELEMENT is a simple substance that cannot be decomposed by ordinary chemical means. An *atom* is the smallest quantity of an element that can exist and still retain the chemical properties of the element. An atom is composed of negatively charged electrons orbiting around a nucleus containing positively charged *protons* and uncharged *neutrons*. The majority of the mass (weight) of an atom exists in its nucleus.

Most elements in their natural state exist with an equal number of positively and negatively charged particles.* An atom is in the *ionized state* when one or more electrons are either removed from or added to the outermost orbit.

Solutions

Many of the important elements in clinical medicine are in solution. A *solution* is a liquid consisting of a mixture of two or more substances that are molecularly dispersed throughout one another in a homogeneous manner. A solution consists of a *solvent* (the major component) and one or more *solutes* (minor components). In biological solutions, water may be considered the major component (solvent); all other substances in solution are considered solutes.

In biological solutions, solutes exist in both un-ionized (undissociated) and ionized (dissociated) states.[8] In other words, that portion of the substance existing in the dissociated state is referred to as an *ion*. It should be obvious that ions have an excess or a deficit of electrons in their outer orbits, that is, ions have net electrical charges. Ions with net positive charges are *cations;* ions with net negative charges are *anions*.

The equilibrium between two states of a substance in solution depends upon several factors, including the chemical interrelationships of the substance and the numbers and types of other substances in the solution (Table 2–1). Certain substances such as strong acids, strong bases, and salts exist in solution primarily in the ionized state. Weak acids and bases exist in solution in varying degrees of ionization.[6] It is

---

*The *atomic number* is based on the number of protons found in the nucleus. The number of protons plus the number of neutrons equals the atomic weight of the atom.

TABLE 2–1.–SUBSTANCES IN SOLUTION

EXAMPLE	UNDISSOCIATED	DISSOCIATED
Strong acid: hydrochloric acid	$HCl \overset{\longrightarrow}{\leftarrow}$	$H^+ + Cl^-$
Strong base: sodium hydroxide	$NaOH \overset{\longrightarrow}{\leftarrow}$	$Na^+ + OH^-$
Salt: sodium chloride	$NaCl \overset{\longrightarrow}{\leftarrow}$	$Na^+ + Cl^-$
Weak acid: carbonic acid	$H_2CO_3 \rightleftharpoons$	$H^+ + HCO_3^-$
Water	$H_2O \overset{\rightarrow}{\longleftarrow}$	$H^+ + OH^-$

important to realize that a small number of water molecules exist in the ionized state.

Hydrogen Ion Activity

The maintenance of cellular function is dependent upon cellular metabolism (biochemical and enzymatic processes).[13] This metabolic process demands an exacting environment. There are many factors, such as temperature, osmolarity, electrolytes, nutrients, and oxygen, that must be maintained within narrow limits if the cell is to preserve its normal metabolic function. One of the most important factors in this cellular environment is the *hydrogen ion activity*—often referred to as the "free hydrogen ion in solution." This is most commonly expressed as *hydrogen ion concentration* ($[H^+]$).

Acids and Bases

Substances that tend to donate hydrogen ions to the solution are called *acids;* substances that tend to remove hydrogen ions from the solution are *bases*.[6] Thus, strong acids are capable of donating many free hydrogen ions to the solution and strong bases can accept many free hydrogen ions from the solution. This situation may be visualized as two points of a spectrum, one end representing a strong acid and the other end representing a strong base. In between these two extremes substances exist that can act as weak acids or weak bases.

Buffers

Weak acids or weak bases will accept or donate hydrogen ions in response to the availability of free hydrogen ions in solution. This phenomenon is extremely important in minimizing changes in free hydrogen ion concentration and thus stabilizing the free hydrogen ion concentration in the cells of biologic systems.[9] A substance that prevents extreme changes in free hydrogen ion concentration within

Buffer Systems

a solution is defined as a *buffer* substance. These buffers allow cellular metabolism to continue unimpeded when the cells are subjected to significant increases or decreases in the number of hydrogen ions. There are four major buffer systems in the body: hemoglobin, bicarbonate, phosphate, and serum protein.[6]

Hb
HCO₃⁻
PO₄
C HbV.

Quantification of Hydrogen Ion Activity

The importance of hydrogen activity in cellular function necessitates its quantitative measurement. The most widely accepted method uses the pH scale. This scale is derived from and dependent upon the fact that water dissociates very weakly to form some hydrogen (H^+) and hydroxyl (OH^-) ions. The relationship can be expressed as an *ionization constant of water* known as a K_W.

$$H_2O \rightleftharpoons H^+ + OH^-$$
$$K_W = \frac{[H^+][OH^-]}{H_2O}$$

Since the concentration of hydrogen and hydroxyl ions is so small, the concentration of undissociated water $[H_2O]$ remains essentially unchanged. Therefore, the K_W of water can be written as follows:

$$K_W = [H^+][OH^-]$$
$$= [1 \times 10^{-7}][1 \times 10^{-7}]$$
$$= 1 \times 10^{-14}$$

Note that an equal number of hydrogen and hydroxyl ions exists, thus the solution is referred to as a *neutral* solution.

Since man is composed of 50–60% water,[13] it is appropriate to use water as the biologic reference solvent. The ionization constant of water (1×10^{-14}) is equal to the product of the concentrations of hydrogen ions and hydroxyl ions; the product of these two concentrations must remain numerically unchanged. Therefore, as hydrogen ions increase in number (an acid solution), there must be a corresponding decrease in the number of hydroxyl ions. Conversely, as hydrogen ions decrease in number (a basic solution), there must be a corresponding increase in the number of hydroxyl ions.[6]

In clinical medicine the emphasis is placed on the hydrogen ion concentration.[13] Because of the small concentrations of hydrogen ion, their expression in the customary fraction or decimal form would be extremely unwieldy. Therefore, an *exponential* form is used to denote the value (Table 2–2). In the exponential form, the power to which 10 must be multiplied is the exponent; for example, in (10^{-3}) the minus

TABLE 2–2.–COMPARISON OF
FRACTION, DECIMAL, AND
EXPONENTIAL FORMS

FRACTION	DECIMAL	EXPONENT
$\frac{1}{10}$	0.1	10^{-1}
$\frac{1}{1,000}$	0.001	10^{-3}
$\frac{1}{10,000,000}$	0.0000001	10^{-7}
$\frac{1}{100,000,000}$	0.00000001	10^{-8}

three (-3) is the exponent. When a number is written in a logarithmic form it can be thought of as a simplified expression of a routine exponential form; 10^{-3} is logarithmically expressed as -3.

At the turn of the century a Scandinavian scientist, S. P. L. Sorenson, who was studying hydrogen ion activity, referred to the concentration 10^{-7} as "7 puissance hydrogen." This is French for describing the hydrogen ion exponent of the base 10 on the logarithmic scale.

The Danish biochemist and physician, Karl Hasselbalch, embraced Sorenson's concept and expressed 10^{-7} mole/L as "the negative logarithm of the hydrogen ion activity." This he called the pH (puissance hydrogen). The mathematical definition of pH is as follows:

$$pH = -\log[H^+]$$

The introduction of a second minus multiplied by the log value allows *all pH values to be expressed as positive numbers* (Table 2–3).

In clinical medicine most blood levels of hydrogen ion concentration lie between 1×10^{-7} mole/L (pH 7) and 1×10^{-8} mole/L (pH 8). The average value for hydrogen ion concentration in blood is 0.4×10^{-8} mole/L (pH 7.4).[6]

TABLE 2–3.–COMPARISON
OF EXPONENTIAL AND
LOGARITHMIC FORMS

EXPONENT	*pH* $(-)$ LOG
10^{-1}	1
10^{-3}	3
10^{-7}	7
10^{-8}	8

Henderson-Hasselbalch Equation

The Henderson-Hasselbalch equation expresses the biologic acid-base relationship by looking at one specific component of the system, namely, the carbonic acid (H_2CO_3) to bicarbonate ion (HCO_3^-) relationship.

$$H_2CO_3 \rightleftharpoons H^+ + HCO_3^- \tag{1}$$

The amount of hydrogen ion activity secondary to the dissociation of carbonic acid is in turn governed by the interrelationship of all the blood acids, bases, and buffers. It is this vital interrelationship that allows for a complete analysis of acid-base balance by looking at only one component of the system.

The *law of mass action* states that in equation (1) the product of the concentrations of the substances on the right divided by the concentration of the substance on the left is equal to a constant written as a value K_A:

$$K_A = \frac{[H^+][HCO_3^-]}{[H_2CO_3]} \tag{2}$$

In order to express the hydrogen ion concentration in pH form, the log of both sides of equation (2) must be taken. This will not change the value of the equation.

$$\log K_A = \log \frac{[H^+][HCO_3^-]}{[H_2CO_3]} \tag{3}$$

$$\log K_A = \log[H^+] + \log \frac{[HCO_3^-]}{[H_2CO_3]} \tag{4}$$

The transposition of the log of the hydrogen ion concentration ($\log[H^+]$) to the left side of equation (4) and the log of K_A to the right side of the equation produces:

$$-\log[H^+] = -\log K_A + \log \frac{[HCO_3^-]}{[H_2CO_3]} \tag{5}$$

The term for minus the log of hydrogen ion concentration ($-\log[H^+]$) has already been defined as pH; the term for minus the log of K_A($-\log K_A$) is the pK.

$$pH = pK + \log \frac{[HCO_3^-]}{[H_2CO_3]} \tag{6}$$

The pK represents the pH value at which the solute is 50% dissociated. In equation (6), if the pH equaled the pK there would be equal amounts of bicarbonate ion and carbonic acid. The importance of the pK is that it represents the pH at which maximum buffering capacity can be achieved for that particular reaction.

In equation (6) the carbonic acid concentration is dependent upon the amount of dissolved carbon dioxide. The amount of carbon dioxide dissolved is in turn dependent upon its solubility (expressed as a solubility coefficient s) and the partial pressure of carbon dioxide measured in the blood (Pco_2). Therefore, in most clinical forms of equation (6), the carbonic acid concentration (H_2CO_3) is replaced by the solubility coefficient times the partial pressure of carbon dioxide ($s \times Pco_2$):

$$pH = pK + \log \frac{[HCO_3^-]}{s \times Pco_2} \tag{7}$$

The pK is 6.1; s is 0.0301.

Carbon Dioxide Chemistry

When carbon dioxide (CO_2) is dissolved in water (dCO_2) the formation of carbonic acid (H_2CO_3) takes place very slowly (Table 2–4). In plasma, the concentration of dissolved carbon dioxide (dCO_2) is approximately 1,000 times greater than the concentration of carbonic acid.

Carbonic Anhydrase

An enzyme is a substance that alters the speed at which a chemical reaction takes place but is not consumed or altered in the process. Carbonic anhydrase is an enzyme that exists in red blood cells and kidney tubular cells. This enzyme speeds the reaction forming carbonic acid (see Table 2–4). Remember, this enzyme does *not* exist in plasma.[6]

TABLE 2–4.– FORMATION OF CARBONIC ACID

Plasma
$$H_2O + dCO_2 \rightarrow H_2CO_3 \rightleftarrows H^+ + HCO_3^-$$
$$1,000 \; : \quad 1$$

Red blood cells
$$H_2O + dCO_2 \rightleftarrows H_2CO_3 \rightleftarrows H^+ + HCO_3^-$$

Total Dissolved Carbon Dioxide

In clinical medicine it is impossible to distinguish between dissolved carbon dioxide (dCO_2) and carbonic acid (H_2CO_3). Therefore, it is convenient to add the respective concentrations and refer to this sum as the *total* dissolved carbon dioxide in plasma.

$$\text{Total } dCO_{2\text{Plasma}} = [dCO_2 + H_2CO_3]_{\text{Plasma}}$$

At BTPS (see Chapter 1) the relationship of this total carbon dioxide dissolved to carbon dioxide partial pressure (PCO_2) can be written as follows:

$$\text{Total carbon dioxide dissolved} = (0.0301)(PCO_2)$$

In other words, the carbon dioxide partial pressure (PCO_2) times its solubility coefficient ($s = 0.0301$) can give the value of the total carbon dioxide dissolved. In essence, a measurement of blood PCO_2 can be considered equivalent to measurement of the plasma carbonic acid plus the dissolved carbon dioxide.

Figure 2–1 illustrates the plasma relationship of dissolved carbon dioxide (dCO_2) and carbonic acid. Most of the carbon dioxide enters the red blood cell, while a small portion remains dissolved in plasma. This small portion is a critical factor that will determine carbon dioxide movement into or out of the blood. As the carbon dioxide tension in cells and extracellular fluid is increased by metabolism, the rate and amount of carbon dioxide movement into the blood are increased.

Fig 2–1.—The plasma relationship of dissolved carbon dioxide (dCO_2) and carbonic acid (H_2CO_3). Note that only a small amount (approximately 5%) of the CO_2 that enters the blood remains in the plasma. Virtually 99.9% of this plasma CO_2 remains in the dissolved state while approximately 0.1% reacts with water to form H_2CO_3, i.e., by volume the relationship of dCO_2/H_2CO_3 is 1,000/1. The dissolved CO_2 exerts a pressure (Henry's law) and is measured clinically as the PCO_2 (partial pressure of carbon dioxide).

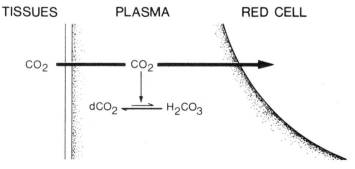

Since carbon dioxide can be dissolved in plasma only to a limited degree, most of the carbon dioxide enters the red blood cells. The red blood cells transport carbon dioxide much more efficiently because of carbonic anhydrase and hemoglobin (see Chapter 3).

In general, the greater the total amount of carbon dioxide in the blood, the greater is the amount present in the plasma (as either dissolved carbon dioxide or carbonic acid). This total dissolved carbon dioxide, although an extremely small portion of the total carbon dioxide content, is extremely critical because it exerts the pressure in the blood that determines the gradient by which carbon dioxide enters or leaves the blood.

3 / Hemoglobin

HEMOGLOBIN is the main component of the red blood cells and is responsible for the red color of blood. A single red blood cell contains approximately 280 million molecules of hemoglobin. Each hemoglobin molecule is approximately 64,500 times the weight of one hydrogen atom and is composed of more than 10,000 atoms of hydrogen, carbon, nitrogen, oxygen, and sulfur. In addition, each hemoglobin molecule contains four atoms of iron—the most significant factor in the ability to carry oxygen. Without hemoglobin, large organisms could neither supply adequate oxygen to their tissues nor transport the carbon dioxide from the tissues to the lungs.

The exact chemical structure of hemoglobin is not entirely known; however, chemical and x-ray analyses have revealed much of the structure and have made even more fascinating the study of this crucial molecule.[15] For those interested in the physiologic process of respiration, an appreciation of this "oxygen carrier" molecule is fundamental.

The Chemistry of Hemoglobin

When four pyrrole rings are cyclically linked through methylene bridges, a *porphyrin* results (Fig 3–1). These porphyrin substances are important in biologic systems primarily because they are capable of forming complexes with metals.[16] A basic theory of chemistry states that chemical compounds may be formed through *covalent bonds.* Covalent bonds are formed between the electrons of two or more atoms. The *ferrous ion* generally has six valence bonds available (Fig 3–2, a). When a ferrous ion (Fe^{++}) binds to a porphyrin ring, each iron atom is attached by covalent bonds to the four nitrogens on the pyrrole groups. The result is a substance known as *heme* (see Fig 3–1).

Amino acids may chemically link to one another to form long chains. Chains of amino acids (polypeptide chains) are known as *protein molecules.* When four specific amino acid chains are combined (two alpha chains and two beta chains), the protein *globin* is the result.[16] This protein molecule contains imidazole nitrogen groups that are capable of forming covalent bonds with metal ions.

Each of the four heme groups in the hemoglobin molecule is believed to be attached to the large protein (globin) by a fifth valence

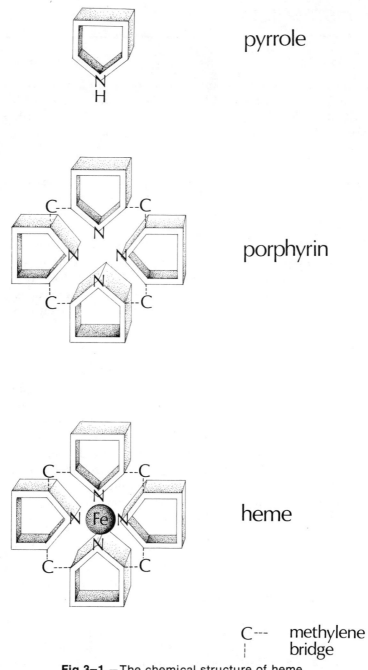

pyrrole

porphyrin

heme

C--- methylene
bridge

Fig 3–1.—The chemical structure of heme.

(a)

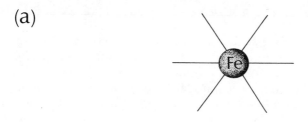

(b)

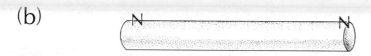

(c)

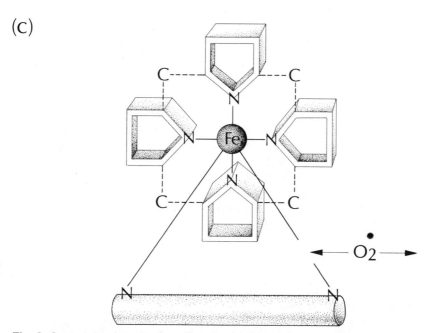

Fig 3–2.—a, the ferrous ion (Fe^{++}) with six potential valence bonds. **b,** schematic representation of a polypeptide chain with two imidazole nitrogens that are capable of forming covalent bonds with metal ions. A protein molecule containing two alpha and two beta polypeptide chains is known as a globin molecule. **c,** heme molecule attached to polypeptide chain. Four heme molecules attached to the four polypeptide chains of a globin molecule comprise the molecule hemoglobin.

bond. In other words, four of the six available ferrous valence bonds are attached to the pyrrole nitrogens; the fifth is attached to globin (see Fig 3–2). *The sixth covalence bond of the iron is available for reversible combination with oxygen.* The linkage of the iron atom in heme to the globin protein confers on the iron the unique power of reacting reversibly with oxygen by means of a neighboring valence bond.

Each of the four atoms of iron in the hemoglobin molecule can reversibly bind to one molecule of oxygen. When this occurs there is a change in color of the hemoglobin; that is, *oxyhemoglobin* (HbO_2) makes arterial blood appear scarlet. Oxygen-free hemoglobin imparts a purplish hue to the blood and is commonly referred to as *reduced hemoglobin* (Hb). The term *reduced* is a misnomer since to the chemist that term means that electrons have been added to an atom or a group of atoms. In fact, the iron atoms in both reduced and oxygenated hemoglobin are in the same electronic condition—the ferrous (Fe^{++}) state. Although chemically incorrect, the term *reduced hemoglobin* is so well established that its use will be retained to delineate the *oxygen-free form of the hemoglobin molecule.*[5]

The Stereochemistry of Hemoglobin

Chemical theory has long recognized the possibility that spatial relationships between molecules and atoms within molecules may affect chemical activity. Few molecules attest to this theory more than the hemoglobin molecule. It is essential to conceive of this large molecule not only in terms of its chemistry but also in terms of its three-dimensional spatial relationships (*stereo*chemistry). Although the stereochemistry of hemoglobin is not completely understood, recent x-ray analyses have elucidated the basics upon which a firm concept may be developed.[17]

Each of the four iron atoms in the hemoglobin molecule lies in the center of the porphyrin ring and is known as heme (see Fig 3–1). In turn, each of the four heme groups is enfolded in one of the four chains of amino acids that collectively constitute the protein portion of the molecule (globin). The four chains contain approximately 574 amino acid units, making it possible for these very large chains to surround and appear to engulf the heme molecules.

Two of the four chains shift back and forth so that the gap between them narrows as oxygen molecules are bound. Conversely, the space between the heme groups widens as oxygen is released from the molecule. This has been described as a "molecular lung" by one of the pioneers in x-ray analysis of the hemoglobin molecule.[17]

Oxygen Affinity

The ability of hemoglobin to reversibly combine with oxygen atoms greatly increases the blood's capability of carrying oxygen from the lungs to the tissues. Thus, delivery of oxygen to the cell depends in good measure upon the *affinity* with which hemoglobin binds and releases oxygen from the red blood cell. The physicochemistry of hemoglobin-oxygen affinity must be understood before the complex physiologic relationships of oxygen transport (see Chapter 9) can be appreciated.

The physicochemical equilibria of hemoglobin with oxygen are only partially delineated at present; however, some generalizations may be safely made if one remembers that they are based upon mathematical theory (primarily Hill's equation and Adair's intermediate compound equation)[16] that has been "adjusted" to more readily explain the observed phenomenon of hemoglobin-oxygen relationships in human red blood cells. Three major factors are presently known to have significant effect on the hemoglobin-oxygen affinity relationships in man: (1) the heme-heme interaction; (2) allosteric interactions; and (3) intra–red blood cell enzyme systems.

Heme-Heme Interaction

Each of the four iron-binding sites in the hemoglobin molecule is affected by the oxygenation status of the other three sites. As each successive heme iron moiety is occupied by oxygen, the distance between them is decreased. These spatial relationships are believed to significantly affect the ability of the unoxygenated heme moieties to combine with oxygen.[17] This physicochemical relationship is probably the basis for the sigmoid shape of the hemoglobin dissociation curve (see Fig 9–3).

Allosteric Interactions

The status of the globin portion of the molecule may affect the spatial relationships of the heme groups. For example, the content of carbon dioxide and hydrogen ion within the red blood cell affects the globin and thereby predictably affects the hemoglobin-oxygen equilibrium.[18] Temperature is believed to affect the mobility and activity of the amino acid chains, thus affecting the heme spatial relationships. The predictable effects of hydrogen ion concentration, carbon dioxide concentration, and temperature on the hemoglobin-oxygen relationship have been known for many years (see Chapter 9).

Red Blood Cell Enzyme Systems

Certain intracellular organic phosphate compounds (e.g., 2,3-diphosphoglycerate) exert profound effects upon the release and binding of oxygen from hemoglobin.[19] These reactions have been only recently described and the full impact of their activity has yet to be determined.[24]

Alteration of Oxygen Affinity

The above three factors are certainly the major physicochemical relationships that affect the *normal* hemoglobin-oxygen equilibria. Numerous conditions are encountered in clinical medicine that alter these equilibria. Of course, any abnormality in the amino acid sequence of the globin chains (hemoglobinopathies) may alter the oxygen affinity. In addition to the hemoglobinopathies, there are three cases so significant that they demand specific consideration: (1) carbon monoxide; (2) methemoglobin; and (3) fetal hemoglobin.

Carbon Monoxide (CO)

Carbon monoxide is capable of forming covalent bonds with the ferrous ion. When this occurs to one or more of the heme groups, *carboxyhemoglobin* (HbCO) is formed. Heme groups combined with carbon monoxide are incapable of combining with oxygen since the carbon monoxide occupies the sixth covalence position.[22]

The affinity of the hemoglobin for carbon monoxide is approximately 200–250 times as great as the affinity for oxygen. The greater the number of heme sites bound to carbon monoxide, the greater is the affinity of the remaining heme sites for oxygen.[20]

In addition, both oxygen and carbon monoxide affinities are affected by the partial pressures of the gases to which the hemoglobin is exposed. Stated simplistically, the greater the partial pressure of oxygen, the less hemoglobin affinity for carbon monoxide; and conversely, the greater the partial pressure of carbon monoxide, the less hemoglobin affinity for oxygen.[21]

Methemoglobin (Met Hb)

Methemoglobin exists when a ferrous ion (Fe^{++}) is oxidized to the ferric (Fe^{+++}) state. This oxidation process causes the hemoglobin to turn a brownish color. Methemoglobin is incapable of combining reversibly with oxygen and thus cannot act as an oxygen carrier.[5] Like carboxyhemoglobin, methemoglobin increases the affinity for oxygen of the remaining iron sites.[10]

Fetal Hemoglobin (HbF)

Fetal hemoglobin comprises approximately 85% of the hemoglobin in the full-term fetus and differs chemically from adult hemoglobin (HbA) in that the two *beta* polypeptide chains are absent and two *gamma* polypeptide chains are present.[23, 24] The gamma chains are believed to affect the physicochemical relationships in such a way that the affinity for oxygen is *increased*.[25, 26] Hemoglobin F is more easily oxidized to methemoglobin than hemoglobin A and there is evidence that the phosphorylase enzyme systems are less active in red blood cells containing hemoglobin F.[27]

Carbon Dioxide Transport

Blood contains both oxygen and carbon dioxide as dissolved gases, i.e., in physical solution. However, of the total amount of these gases present in the blood, almost all the gas exists in reversible chemical combination rather than in physical solution. In other words, oxygen is "carried" or "transported" by direct chemical combination with hemoglobin.

Carbon dioxide is also carried by direct chemical combination with hemoglobin, but the red blood cell's capability of rapidly producing bicarbonate ion constitutes a second major transport system. Thus, the two major carbon dioxide transport mechanisms in the blood are: (1) the carbamino mechanism and (2) the bicarbonate ion mechanism.

Carbamino-CO_2 Mechanism

Carbamino compounds are formed when carbon dioxide chemically combines with amino acids. While only a fraction of the carbon dioxide entering the red blood cell combines directly with hemoglobin, it is the *difference* in the quantity of this substance in reduced and oxygenated hemoglobin that plays a significant role in CO_2 transport.[28] For resting man at sea level, it has been estimated that 20–30% of the *change* in the carbon dioxide content of whole blood is due to carbamino-CO_2.[29] Thus, it is reasonable to conceive of this mechanism as being responsible for 20–30% of the blood's CO_2 transport capabilities.[6]

Bicarbonate Ion Mechanism

Red blood cells and kidney tubular cells contain the enzyme *carbonic anhydrase*.[30] An enzyme is generally defined as a protein substance that speeds specific chemical reactions. The presence of carbonic anhydrase (CA) speeds the hydrating reaction of carbon dioxide to form carbonic acid:

$$CO_2 + H_2O \xrightarrow[CA]{} H_2CO_3 \longrightarrow H^+ + HCO_3^-$$

The presence of carbonic anhydrase enables the red blood cells to carry carbon dioxide efficiently because carbonic acid is rapidly dissociated into hydrogen and bicarbonate ions. Since hemoglobin is an excellent buffer (see Chapter 2) it allows great changes in hydrogen ion content to occur while minimizing the changes in free hydrogen ions (pH).

As carbon dioxide enters the blood (Fig 3–3), a small amount remains in physical solution in the plasma (see Chapter 2) while the remainder enters the red blood cell. A portion of this carbon dioxide attaches directly to the hemoglobin to form carbamino-CO_2, while approximately 65% of the carbon dioxide is rapidly transformed to hydrogen and bicarbonate ions. The hydrogen ions are chemically bound to the hemoglobin.

Bicarbonate ions diffuse into the plasma because the *red blood cell to plasma gradient* becomes greater as the carbon dioxide content of

Fig 3–3.—A schematic representation of carbon dioxide transport in blood (see text). Note that only a small portion of plasma bicarbonate (HCO_3^-) is determined by this mechanism; the great majority of the plasma bicarbonate is determined by renal (kidney) mechanisms.

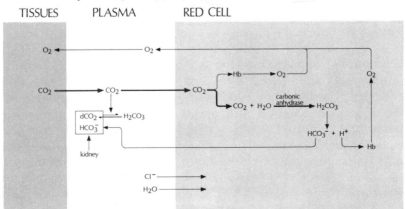

the blood increases. Thus, as bicarbonate leaves the red blood cell, the laws of electrostatics result in the chloride ion migrating into the red blood cell in order to maintain electrical neutrality. This decrease in plasma chloride concentration secondary to increased bicarbonate ion concentration is known as the *chloride shift.*

As the carbon dioxide content of blood increases there is a corresponding increase in osmotically active particles within the red blood cells. Thus water tends to move from plasma into the erythrocytes, causing them to swell slightly as arterial blood becomes venous.

Oxygen and Carbon Dioxide Interaction

Bohr first described the underlying chemical factor governing the hemoglobin molecule's reaction to oxygen and CO_2: *Oxygenated hemoglobin is a stronger acid than deoxygenated hemoglobin.*[31] In simplistic terms, this chemical observation means that as arterial (oxygenated) blood begins to give up oxygen to the tissues, the loss of oxygen from the hemoglobin makes the molecule a weaker acid (i.e., more capable of binding with hydrogen ions). This phenomenon obviously increases the blood's ability to transport the carbon dioxide which is entering the blood at this time. Conversely, as the blood passes through the lungs, the oxygenation of the hemoglobin makes it a stronger acid (i.e., less capable of binding with hydrogen ion). This phenomenon obviously aids the reversal of the bicarbonate ion and carbamino mechanisms, allowing carbon dioxide to be reformed and excreted through the lungs as the blood is oxygenated.

The effects of Bohr's observation have been used over the years to describe the intricacies of the interrelationships of oxygen and CO_2 transport mechanisms as they relate to hemoglobin. The so-called *Bohr effect* most commonly refers to the phenomenon that the addition of carbon dioxide to the blood will enhance oxygen release from hemoglobin. The *Haldane effect* most commonly refers to the phenomenon that the addition of oxygen to the blood will enhance the release of carbon dioxide from the hemoglobin.[32]

Obviously, these are simply alternative ways to describe the chemical interrelationships of oxygen, CO_2, and the hemoglobin molecule. From a chemical viewpoint it is reasonable to state that the effect of oxygenation on carbon dioxide transport is several times more important than the effect of carbon dioxide on oxygen transport.[16]

4 / Physics and Chemistry of Blood Gas Measurement

THE MEASUREMENT of blood pH, PCO_2 and PO_2 is accomplished by specially designed electrodes, the understanding of which depends upon a knowledge of basic electrical physics. In essence, the flow of electrons from one point to another is referred to as an electric *current*. Such an electron flow occurs in response to a *potential difference* between two points in a manner similar to a gas flowing in response to a pressure difference between two points. An electrical potential difference *(voltage)* is measured by devices called *voltmeters*. An electrical device that can predictably vary potential differences (voltage) is called a *potentiometer*.

pH Electrode

It was discovered more than fifty years ago that if two solutions of different pHs are separated by a particular type of glass membrane, a potential difference will exist across the "pH-sensitive" glass.[33-37] As shown in Figure 4–1, a, if a solution of known pH (6.840) is separated by pH-sensitive glass from a solution of unknown pH, a measurable voltage will be developed across the glass.

Chemical half-cells (Fig 4–1, b) are used to accurately measure the small potential differences accompanying blood pH variations.[38] The *reference electrode* is usually composed of mercury-mercurous chloride (calomel)—a substance that supplies a constant reference voltage as long as the temperature remains stable.[37] The *measuring electrode* is usually composed of a silver-silver chloride substance whose function is to convey the potential difference existing across the glass membrane to the electronic circuitry.[37]

Modern Electrode

The modern pH electrode (Fig 4–1, c) has the measuring half-cell imbedded within a 6.840 buffer chamber. This half-cell and the adjacent sampling chamber are encased in a constant-temperature water bath. The reference half-cell is electronically connected to the measuring half-cell by a *contact bridge*—a potassium chloride (KCl) solution that completes the electronic circuit. The blood (unknown solu-

(a)

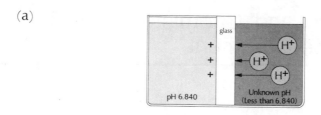

(b)

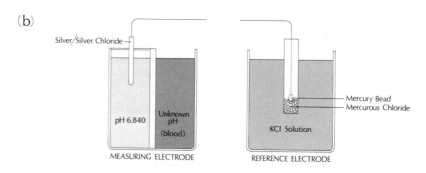

(c)

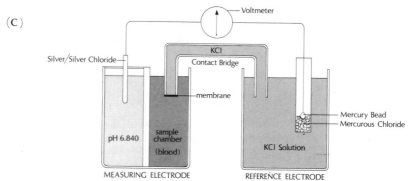

Fig 4–1.—Basic principles of the pH electrode. **a,** voltage developed across pH-sensitive glass when hydrogen ion concentration is unequal in the two solutions. **b,** chemical half-cell is used as the measuring electrode and another half-cell is the reference electrode (see text). **c,** the basic principle of the modern pH electrode (see text).

tion) is separated from the salt (KCl) solution by a membrane so that contamination cannot occur.

Calibration

The relationships between the potential difference $(E_u - E_k)$ and the pHs of the known (pH_k) and unknown (pH_u) solutions are defined by the modified Nernst equation:[37]

$$pH_u = pH_k + \left(\frac{E_u - E_k}{2.3026T}\right)\left(\frac{F}{R}\right)$$

Where R is the molar gas constant, F is the Faraday constant, and T is the absolute temperature. If the pH of the unknown solution is equal to that of the known solution, the potential difference $(E_u - E_k)$ will be zero. A potential of 61.5 millivolts (mv) will be developed for every pH unit difference between the two solutions at 37°C.[39]

Potentiometers convert the potential differences to the correct pH scale readout. When 6.840 buffer solution is in the measuring half-cell, the potential difference is zero and the electronic display is set to 6.840 by a *balance potentiometer*. When the measuring half-cell is filled with 7.384 buffer solution, the difference between the two half-cells is 0.544 pH units, and a 33.5 mv potential difference can be predicted. Thus, the voltmeter will measure 33.5 mv and a *slope potentiometer* sets the electronic display at 7.384. Since the potential difference is a linear function of the pH, two-point calibration is usually sufficient for accurate blood pH measurement.

Sanz Electrode

A clinical system for pH measurement must meet several demands before it can be considered practical and applicable: (1) the blood sample must remain anaerobic; (2) the measuring cycle must require a minimal volume of blood; and (3) a constant temperature must be maintained. Figure 4–2 illustrates the typical design of a modern, ultramicro pH electrode first developed in the mid 1950s and most often referred to as the Sanz electrode.[40] The pH-sensitive glass has been rolled into a fine capillary tube, allowing the necessary blood volume to be as little as 25 microliters (μl) and remain anaerobic.[41] The entire electrode is small enough to be contained in a thermostatically controlled environment in order to assure a constant temperature.[42-44]

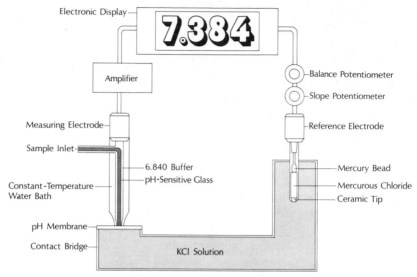

Fig 4–2.—Schematic illustration of the modern, ultramicro pH electrode (see text).

Pco₂ Electrode

Henry's law (see Chapter 1) states that the amount of gas diffusing across a permeable membrane is directly proportional to the pressure gradient. As shown in Figure 4–3, if a carbon dioxide partial pressure gradient exists across a permeable membrane with an aqueous bicarbonate solution on the other side, carbon dioxide entering the solution undergoes the following chemical reaction[45]:

$$CO_2 + H_2O \rightarrow H_2CO_3 \rightarrow H^+ + HCO_3^-$$

The hydrogen ion concentration developed is directly proportional to the Pco₂ in contact with the membrane.[46] Utilizing the aqueous bicarbonate chamber as the measuring half-cell, the pH change can be measured and utilized as an indirect measure of the Pco₂ of the blood.

Fig 4–3.—Basic principle of the Pco₂ electrode (see text). The *shaded area* represents an aqueous bicarbonate solution.

GASEOUS CO₂ ⟶ $CO_2 + H_2O \rightleftharpoons H_2CO_3 \rightleftharpoons H^+ + HCO_3^-$

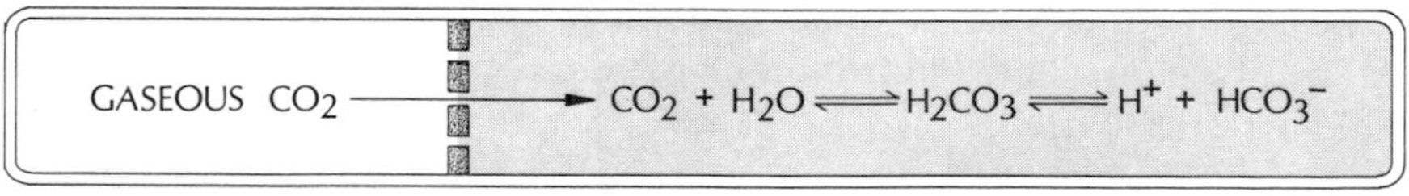

Modern Electrode

A silicon elastic membrane separates the blood sample from the measuring half-cell (Fig 4–4).[47] The pH-sensitive glass is separated from the membrane by a nylon spacer that allows an aqueous bicarbonate solution (electrolyte) to exist between the glass and the permeable membrane. The measuring half-cell is silver-silver chloride; the reference half-cell is another silver-silver chloride unit rather than calomel.[48,49]

The entire electrode is in a lucite jacket and is bathed in electrolyte solution. This electrolyte constantly replenishes the solution at the electrode tip and provides an electric contact bridge between the measuring and reference half-cells.

Calibration

Gases analyzed to precise concentrations are used to calibrate the Pco_2 electrode.[50] A gas mixture with a CO_2 concentration of 5% is commonly chosen as the balance point, and a slope point is set with a gas having approximately 10% CO_2 concentration. The Pco_2 will be directly proportional to the hydrogen ion concentration as measured by the pH electrode system.[51]

Severinghaus Electrode

Until the mid 1950s, methods used to measure Pco_2 were cumbersome and time consuming.[52,53] Some involved the direct measurement of pH and carbon dioxide content—the Henderson-Hasselbalch equation (see Chapter 2) was then used to extrapolate the Pco_2.[54] Another popular method in the 1940s and 1950s was known as the "CO_2-com-

Fig 4–4.—Schematic illustration of the modern Pco_2 electrode (see text). The space between the silicon membrane and the nylon spacer is greatly enlarged for clarity.

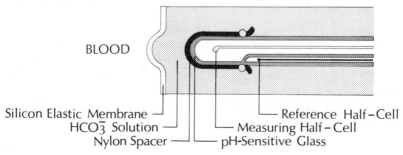

BLOOD

Silicon Elastic Membrane ⏤
HCO₃⁻ Solution ⏤
Nylon Spacer ⏤
Reference Half–Cell
Measuring Half–Cell
pH-Sensitive Glass

bining power," which involved the equilibration between blood and a bubble of gas having a known carbon dioxide content. By measuring the carbon dioxide content after equilibration, the P_{CO_2} was extrapolated.[55]

The modern P_{CO_2} electrode was first introduced by Stowe[56] and was further modified by Severinghaus in 1958.[57] This electrode is commonly referred to as the *Severinghaus electrode.*

Po_2 Electrode

Gaining electrons in a chemical reaction is known as *reduction* and occurs at a cathode; the loss of electrons in a chemical reaction is known as *oxidation* and occurs at an anode. If oxygen is dissolved in an aqueous medium and exposed to a polarizing voltage at a cathode, the following reaction occurs:

$$O_2 + 2H_2O + 4 \text{ electrons } (e^-) \rightarrow 4 \text{ OH}^-$$

This chemical reduction of oxygen is the principle of the polarographic electrode.[58]

The Polarographic Electrode

A silver anode immersed in a potassium chloride electrolyte solution will attract chloride anions (Cl^-) to form silver chloride (Fig 4–5). This oxidation reaction produces a constant flow of electrons (current). An adjacent platinum cathode will react chemically with oxygen to form hydroxyl ions (OH^-)—a reduction reaction that uses electrons. In general, as electrons are consumed at the cathode, the anode reaction is accelerated.

Figure 4–5 illustrates that the amount of oxygen reduced will be directly proportional to the number of electrons used in the cathode reaction. Thus, by measuring the change in current (electron flow) between the anode and the cathode, the amount of oxygen in the electrode solution can be determined.

An external polarizing voltage of −0.6 volt is required to minimize the interference of other gases that can also be reduced and to assure rapid oxygen reduction at the cathode. Thus, the common electrical concept of an anode as a negative electrode and a cathode as a positive electrode is not applicable.[58] However, the chemical definition of a cathode as the reduction pole and the anode as the oxidation pole remains unchanged.

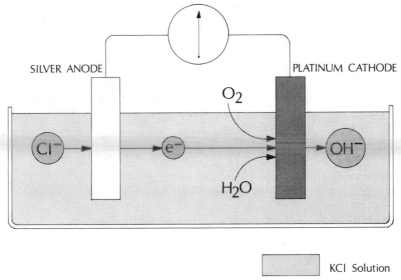

KCl Solution

Fig 4–5.—The basic principle of the polarographic electrode. The chloride ion will react with the silver anode to form silver chloride—an oxidation reaction that produces electrons. Oxygen will react with platinum and water utilizing electrons (a reduction reaction). The flow of electrons can be measured as a current. The greater the concentration of oxygen in solution, the greater the current used (see text).

Calibration

An analyzed gas mixture with an oxygen concentration of 0% is selected as the balance point; the slope point is set with a gas having either 12% or 20% oxygen. For convenience and economy, the calibration gases for the PO_2 and PCO_2 electrodes are combined. One gas is usually composed of 5% CO_2 and 12% or 20% O_2, with the remainder composed of nitrogen; the second gas is usually 10% CO_2 and 90% N_2.

The Clark Electrode

The entire electrode system is usually covered by a polypropylene membrane, which allows a slow diffusion of oxygen from the blood into the electrode (Fig 4–6).[59] A slow-diffusing membrane is selected to prevent depletion of oxygen while the measurement is taking place.[60,61] This negates the need for stirring the blood and significantly decreases electrode instability.[62]

P$_{O_2}$ ELECTRODE:

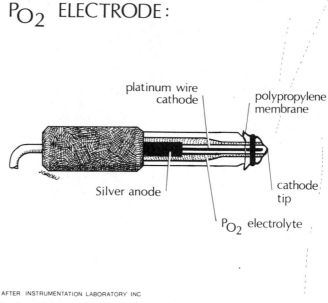

platinum wire cathode

polypropylene membrane

Silver anode

cathode tip

P$_{O_2}$ electrolyte

AFTER INSTRUMENTATION LABORATORY INC

Fig 4–6. — Schematic illustration of the Clark electrode (see text).

Although the first polarographic oxygen electrodes were developed in the late 1930s,[63,64] the development of the modern electrode in the 1950s for measuring blood and other solutions is attributed to Clark.[65] For this reason the P$_{O_2}$ electrode is commonly referred to as the *Clark electrode.*

The Galvanic Electrode

The principle of operation of the galvanic electrode is similar to the Clark electrode except that the galvanic cell produces *internally* the voltage for the cathode reduction.[58] In other words, as oxygen enters the cell across a plastic membrane, electron production begins at the anode. This reaction is essentially irreversible, making the life of the electrode dependent upon the concentration and duration of oxygen exposure.

The cathode is usually composed of gold, the anode of lead, and the electrolyte solution is potassium hydroxide. The entire cathode is sealed and has a permanent membrane covering the large cathode surface.[66]

The Modern Blood Gas Analyzer

The past fifteen years have seen the development of several machines capable of measuring pH, P_{CO_2}, and P_{O_2} reliably and accurately. Their costs are within the budgets of most hospitals and a well-trained laboratory technician or respiratory therapist has the skills needed for proper operation. This technology has been adequately applied by several manufacturers to make the modern blood gas analyzer a clinical reality. Although there are numerous differences between the various models, all the analyzers contain the following three electrodes.

The Sanz (pH) electrode quantifies the relative acidity and alkalinity of a blood solution by measuring the potential difference across a pH-sensitive glass membrane. Its principle of operation is related to the measurement of voltages and therefore the electrode is referred to as *potentiometric*.[58]

The Severinghaus (P_{CO_2}) electrode measures carbon dioxide tensions by allowing the carbon dioxide gas to undergo a chemical reaction to produce hydrogen ions. The hydrogen ion concentration is measured by half-cells similar to the Sanz electrode. This system is also *potentiometric*.

The Clark (P_{O_2}) electrode measures oxygen by electron consumption. The electron flow is measured in amperage and is referred to as *amperometric*.[58]

The precision of these measurements is dependent upon many things, but the ability to maintain the electrodes at a constant temperature is a prominent factor. This is accomplished by enclosing the electrodes in thermostatically controlled water baths or heating blocks.[42-44]

Spectrophotometry

In addition to pH, P_{CO_2}, and P_{O_2} measurements, it is desirable to measure hemoglobin content (see Chapter 9) and the percentage of oxyhemoglobin present in the blood. The most popular method for such measurements is spectrophotometry, the understanding of which is dependent upon a knowledge of the basic physics of light.

Basic Physics of Light

Light is an electromagnetic form of energy. The physical properties of light are characterized by a *wavelength* and a *frequency*, which have fixed relationships with one another. The energy properties of light are referred to as separate energy "packets" known as *quanta.* Thus, the *intensity* of a beam of light refers to the number of quanta generated per second.[67]

The atoms in any molecule are constantly vibrating; the vibrations are similar to the vibrations generated by light waves. In general, *light passing through a substance that has the same frequency as the vibrations between the atoms of that substance will tend to be absorbed.* A particular molecule's vibrational characteristics can be drawn as a *spectrum,* that is, a graph of a molecule's absorbance of electromagnetic energies at various wavelengths.

The Spectrophotometer

A spectrophotometer generates light at a known intensity going into a solution, and measures the intensity of light leaving the solution (Fig 4-7). If that light source has wavelengths in sympathy with the vibrational frequencies of certain molecules in the solution, the concentration of those molecules can be measured. The principle of this measurement is that the intensity of light that is absorbed while passing through the solution will be proportional to the concentration of that molecule within the solution (Beer's law).

The Oximeter

The hemoglobin molecule exists in various forms, e.g., oxy-, reduced, carboxy-, sulf-, met-, and fetal (see Chapter 3). Each of these forms has its own light spectrum.[68] A spectrophotometer with specific wavelengths for the oxyhemoglobin spectrum is called an *oximeter.* Therefore, an oximeter is a device for determining the concentration of oxyhemoglobin in blood.

Fig 4–7.—Basic principle of the spectrophotometer (see text).

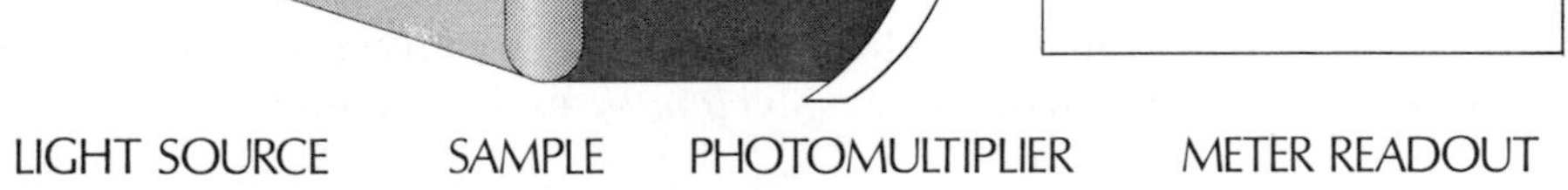

LIGHT SOURCE   SAMPLE   PHOTOMULTIPLIER   METER READOUT

The CO-Oximeter

Instrumentation Laboratory, Inc.,* has developed and marketed a spectrophotometer capable of simultaneously analyzing three spectra—reduced hemoglobin, oxyhemoglobin, and carboxyhemoglobin.[69, 70] This CO-Oximeter makes these three measurements and reports the sum as the hemoglobin concentration in grams per 100 milliliters; the oxyhemoglobin and carboxyhemoglobin are reported as percents of the hemoglobin concentration.[71]

---

*Lexington, MA 02173.

SECTION II

The Physiology of Respiration

BLOOD OXYGEN AND CARBON DIOXIDE exist partially in dissolved form and as such exert pressure. The measurement of the partial pressures exerted by these gases may be called *blood gas measurement*. Although hydrogen is not normally present in the blood as a gas, the determination of blood pH has become an automatic and universally accepted companion of P_{CO_2} and P_{O_2} measurement. *This book will consider the blood gases as the measurement of P_{O_2}, P_{CO_2}, and pH.*

Pulmonary function studies are concerned with ventilation—the mass movement of air into and out of the lungs. Blood gas studies are concerned with *respiration*—the exchange of gases between air and blood and between blood and tissue. Blood gas results have clinical significance only in relation to the efficiency or inefficiency with which several organ systems meet the metabolic demands. In the care of the critically ill, the ability to properly interpret arterial blood gases is essential. In respiratory care, whether one is dealing with critically ill patients or not, the proper use of arterial blood gas measurements is an absolute clinical necessity.

The previous section considered the basic chemistry and physics necessary to comprehend the physiology related to the blood gases. The following seven chapters discuss the basic physiology of the cardiopulmonary homeostatic schema and the physiology related to each of the three blood gas measurements. The reader must appreciate that only the material considered essential for intelligent clinical application of the measurements is discussed. By no means are the following chapters intended to be a complete presentation of respiratory physiology.

5 / Cardiopulmonary Homeostasis

> *Homeostasis* . . . the tendency of a system,
> esp. the physiological system of higher
> animals, to maintain internal stability, owing to
> the coordinated response of its parts to any
> situation or stimulus tending to disturb its
> normal condition or function. — *The Random
> House Dictionary of the English Language*

THE SINGLE-CELLED ANIMAL very simply acquires oxygen from the environment and expels the carbon dioxide metabolite; the entire process requires nothing more than simple diffusion across the cell membrane. In man, the homeostatic necessity of gas exchange (respiration) involves the cardiopulmonary system—two distinct sets of capillary beds plus the pulmonary and cardiovascular systems.

Cardiopulmonary homeostasis may be conceived as the resultant of the mechanisms acting upon the cardiovascular and pulmonary systems to maintain adequate respiration. Figure 5–1 illustrates many of the components of this delicate balance. One must comprehend the primary factors that determine cardiopulmonary homeostasis because *it is this homeostasis that the blood gases reflect.*

Systemic Capillary System

At the distal end of the systemic arterial system is the *systemic capillary bed,* which pervades nearly all tissues. This is where gas exchange between blood and tissue takes place—the exchange known as *internal respiration.* It is measured by the *respiratory quotient,* which is the ratio of the carbon dioxide produced to the oxygen consumed. The normal value of the respiratory quotient is 0.8.

Gas exchange in the systemic capillary bed depends on many factors, including:
1. Values of arterial blood gases entering the capillary bed.
2. Blood distribution throughout the capillary bed.
3. Arterial-to-venous shunting; i.e., the bypassing of the capillaries.
4. Rate of blood flow through the capillary bed.
5. Cardiac output, i.e., the total amount of blood circulated per minute.

EXTERNAL RESPIRATION

PULMONARY CAPILLARY BED
R.R. = 0.8

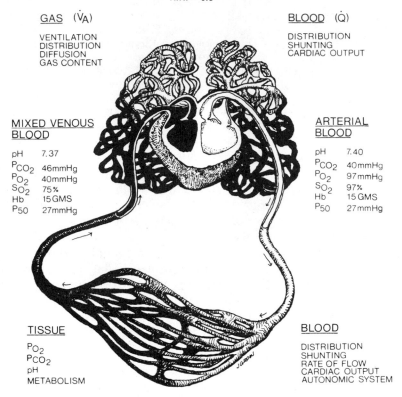

GAS ($\dot{V}_A$)

VENTILATION
DISTRIBUTION
DIFFUSION
GAS CONTENT

BLOOD ($\dot{Q}$)

DISTRIBUTION
SHUNTING
CARDIAC OUTPUT

MIXED VENOUS
BLOOD

pH	7.37
P_{CO_2}	46mmHg
P_{O_2}	40mmHg
S_{O_2}	75%
Hb	15GMS
P_{50}	27mmHg

ARTERIAL
BLOOD

pH	7.40
P_{CO_2}	40mmHg
P_{O_2}	97mmHg
S_{O_2}	97%
Hb	15GMS
P_{50}	27mmHg

TISSUE

P_{O_2}
P_{CO_2}
pH
METABOLISM

BLOOD

DISTRIBUTION
SHUNTING
RATE OF FLOW
CARDIAC OUTPUT
AUTONOMIC SYSTEM

R.Q. = 0.8
SYSTEMIC CAPILLARY BED

INTERNAL RESPIRATION

Fig 5–1.—The cardiopulmonary homeostatic schema (see text).

  6. Autonomic nervous system effects on the capillaries.
  7. Tissue oxygen tension.
  8. Tissue carbon dioxide tension.
  9. Tissue pH.
 10. Metabolic rate.

If one or more of these factors are abnormal, the homeostatic cycle
will be affected.

Pulmonary Capillary System

Blood entering into a portion of the systemic venous system reflects only the gas exchange of that particular tissue and may have inconsistent relationships with the total body homeostasis; total body homeostatic reflection is possible after venous blood mixes in the right ventricle. The mixed venous blood (pulmonary artery blood) enters the *pumonary capillary bed* (in the lungs), where gas exchange between blood and atmosphere takes place. This exchange of oxygen and carbon dioxide, known as *external respiration,* is measured by the respiratory exchange ratio (RR).[72] This ratio (approximately 0.8) is numerically very close to the respiratory quotient (RQ) since external and internal respiration are equal in the steady state.

The factors involved in gas exchange in the pulmonary capillary bed include:
1. Distribution of the blood flow.
2. Intrapulmonary shunting.
3. Cardiac output.
4. Total ventilation (air movement into and out of the airway).
5. Distribution of inspired gases throughout the tracheobronchial tree and the alveoli.
6. Diffusion across the alveolar-capillary membrane.
7. Content of the inspired air.

Arterial Versus Venous Blood

It should be obvious that venous blood collected from the systemic and pulmonary capillary beds, respectively, is mixed together in the corresponding ventricles. Thus, blood leaving those ventricles must be measured if reflection of total body gas exchange is desired. Since respiration does not occur in the arteries, any arterial blood sample represents blood leaving the corresponding ventricle. The easy availability of systemic arteries has made them the universal standard for obtaining clinical blood gas samples.

Homeostatic Balance and Blood Gases

A change of any factor in the cardiopulmonary homeostatic schema (see Fig 5–1) results in either: (1) the arterial blood gas values changing, or (2) an organ system increasing its work to maintain the

homeostatic balance—the blood gas values remain relatively unchanged; or (3) various combinations of these two alternatives.

The degree of abnormality found in arterial blood gas measurement
is determined by the balance between the severity of disease and the
degree of compensation (increased work) by the cardiopulmonary system. *Normal arterial blood gases do NOT mean there is an absence of
cardiopulmonary disease:* there may be disease present but totally
compensated. *Abnormal arterial blood gases mean that uncompensated disease is present*—a situation that may be life threatening.

6 / The Physiology of Internal Respiration

THE PRIMARY BIOLOGIC PURPOSE of respiration is to provide oxygen to the cells; the secondary purpose is to remove carbon dioxide from the cells. *Tissue oxygenation may be considered the primary purpose of internal respiration* — the process of molecular gas exchange at the blood-tissue interface. This process is essential for normal cellular metabolism; in essence, oxygen is consumed and carbon dioxide is produced.

The process of tissue oxygenation involves many factors. Table 6–1 outlines the major factors and denotes the chapters in which they are discussed.

Cellular Oxygen

As the earth's atmosphere developed from containing primarily hydrogen (a reducing atmosphere) to containing primarily oxygen (an oxidizing atmosphere), oxygen became available as an energy source for the development of cellular life because it was abundant, accessible, and possessed a high energy potential. Thus, life forms developed using oxygen as the primary biomedical storage type of energy; in fact, complex forms of life evolved only after mechanisms for maintaining the cellular oxygen environment were developed.

The transition to an oxygen atmosphere forced complex biologic systems to develop defenses against the toxic effects of oxygen. These toxic effects of oxygen were first alluded to by the discoverers of oxygen. In 1785 Lavoisier noted that oxygen must be considered a biomedical double-edged sword — it not only promotes life but also destroys life.[73] He noted that when there is an excess of oxygen, an animal undergoes a severe illness; when oxygen is lacking, death is almost instantaneous.

We now understand that increasing the oxygen tension in tissues will increase the energy available for biologic processes. However, more of the cellular constituents will be destroyed as oxygen tension increases. These two effects occur at all concentrations of oxygen and, thus, *there must be an oxygen pressure at which biologic activity is optimal.*[74,75] If the oxygen tension is significantly above or below this optimal pressure, there are dire biologic consequences.

47

TABLE 6–1.–MAJOR FACTORS IN TISSUE OXYGENATION

SUBJECT	CHAPTER
A. Cellular oxygen utilization	6
Tissue hypoxia	
Metabolic rate	
B. Cellular oxygen delivery	6
Heart Function	
Systemic vascular system	
Microcirculatory system	
C. Aterial oxygen content	9
Arterial oxygenation	
Hemoglobin oxygenation	
D. External respiration	7, 8, 9

Cellular energy is necessary for chemical reactions. Many essential biochemical reactions for sustaining life require a considerable amount of energy, in fact, so much energy that they have been referred to as "thermodynamically improbable." This means that the energy required for many necessary biochemical cellular functions is so great that it is almost impossible for the cell to manufacture such energy. The cell obtains this great amount of energy from substances called *high-energy phosphate bonds*, primarily the high-energy phosphate bonds contained in adenosine triphosphate (ATP). Most cellular energy is utilized, transported, and stored in the form of these high-energy phosphate bonds. Breakdown of these bonds is accompanied by a tremendous energy release.[76]

Oxidative metabolism is the normal mechanism by which energy is stored and released from high-energy phosphate bonds. The *mitochondria* are cellular constituents that contain all the components necessary to form and break down ATP. Molecular oxygen must be available in the cell in order for the biochemical process within the mitochondria (Krebs cycle) to produce high-energy phosphate bonds and allow the release of energy for biochemical processes.[76]

When the delivery of oxygen to the mitochondria is impaired, the energy contained within the Krebs cycle is no longer available. The cellular oxygen tension at which the mitochondrial respiratory rate begins to decrease is called the *critical oxygen tension*.[76] Various studies show that as long as other factors are normal, the mitochondria can function adequately when cellular oxygen tension is less than 5 mm Hg.[76] At the present time, however, it is not possible to delineate critical oxygen tensions for vital organ systems under various conditions.

Tissue Hypoxia

Tissue hypoxia exists when cellular critical oxygen tensions are inadequate. This statement seems clinically appropriate since the importance of tissue hypoxia is that mechanisms other than oxidative ones must be used to provide metabolic energy. These *anaerobic* mechanisms are homeostatically undesirable because they are far less efficient than aerobic pathways and they produce metabolites other than carbon dioxide.

Classically, hypoxia is subdivided into four types: (1) hypoxemic hypoxia (anoxic anoxia); (2) anemic hypoxia (anemic anoxia); (3) circulatory hypoxia (circulatory anoxia); and (4) histotoxic hypoxia. These may be summarized in the following manner.

Hypoxemic Hypoxia

This is deficient tissue oxygenation due to an inadequate arterial blood oxygen tension (hypoxemia). The hemoglobin available is insufficiently oxygenated and the resulting oxygen content is inadequate to maintain an adequate blood to tissue oxygen tension gradient (see Chapter 9). *In essence this is hypoxia due to hypoxemia!* However, the presence of arterial hypoxemia does not automatically indicate the presence of tissue hypoxia, since the cardiovascular system may adequately compensate by increasing cardiac output so that less oxygen is removed from each given quantity of blood. This mechanism frequently allows tissue oxygen requirements to be met (see Chapter 9). It should be emphasized that although hypoxemia does not necessarily indicate that tissue hypoxia is present, it must strongly *suggest* tissue hypoxia and necessitates complete clinical evaluation.

Anemic Hypoxia

This represents deficient tissue oxygenation because of a reduction in the oxygen-carrying capacity of the blood, that is, a deficiency either in the amount of hemoglobin present (anemia) or in the ability of the hemoglobin to carry oxygen (methemoglobinemia, carbon monoxide poisoning, and others). *The arterial blood may have a perfectly normal arterial oxygen tension.* This is one of the circumstances that stress the importance for the clinician to realize the difference between arterial oxygen tension and arterial oxygen content (see Chapter 9).

The main compensatory mechanism for anemic hypoxia is an increase in cardiac output (see Chapter 9). As a general statement it can be said that anemic hypoxia is rarely accompanied by hypoxemia.

Circulatory Hypoxia

Capillary circulation may become inadequate to meet the cellular requirement of oxygen. This can be thought of as either capillary stagnation (pooling) of the blood or failure of the capillaries to allow a flow of blood to the tissues (arterial-venous shunting).

Stagnant hypoxia is the result of a sluggish peripheral capillary blood flow, which may be caused by decreased cardiac output, vascular insufficiency, or neurochemical abnormalities. The slow transit time of the blood through the capillaries results in prolonged oxygen exchange between a given amount of capillary blood and tissues. This exchange is eventually limited by an inadequate blood to tissue oxygen pressure gradient. Since tissue metabolism continues, a decrease in tissue oxygen tension (hypoxia) results. Stagnant hypoxia is primarily a cardiovascular phenomenon and commonly occurs unassociated with arterial hypoxemia (see Chapter 9); however, it is almost always associated with a severe reduction in venous oxygen content and venous oxygen tension (see Chapter 20).

Certain clinical conditions (e.g., sepsis) lead to *arterial-venous shunting* in the systemic capillaries. Where this occurs, capillary blood flow is absent and therefore oxygen is unavailable to the tissues. Often this type of tissue hypoxia is associated with above-normal cardiac outputs and is not associated with decreased arterial and venous oxygen tensions.

Histotoxic Hypoxia

This represents tissue oxygen deficiency due to failure of oxygen utilization at the cellular level. It is rarely accompanied by hypoxemia. The classic example is cyanide poisoning but it has also been reported in alcohol poisoning.

Summary

Tissue hypoxia is the condition in which inadequate oxygen is available at the cellular level. Its direct measurement is not available and therefore it remains a purely clinical diagnosis. The condition is presumed from various clinical and laboratory findings. In clinical medicine, total cellular oxygen utilization is conceived as the metabolic rate or, more specifically, the total oxygen consumption.

Metabolic Rate

The basilar oxygen consumption of an average-size adult is approximately 250 ml/min.[8] Aerobic metabolism produces 80 ml carbon dioxide for each 100 ml oxygen consumed; this respiratory quotient (RQ) of 0.8 means that the normal adult male will produce 200 ml carbon dioxide for each 250 ml oxygen consumed.[12] Increases in metabolic rate can occur suddenly (such as in exercise)[3] or they can gradually increase over periods of minutes to hours (such as a slow rise in a patient's temperature).[9] An *increase* in body temperature is the most common reason for a change in metabolic rate. Fever is responsible for a 10% increase in oxygen consumption for each degree Celsius (centigrade) rise in temperature (7% increase per degree Fahrenheit).[8] Sudden increases in metabolic rate can be seen in patients who have had a grand mal seizure or a sudden increase in the work of breathing, such as would occur secondary to a partial upper airway obstruction. However, *under normal clinical circumstances the moment-to-moment demand for oxygen at the tissue level is fairly constant.*

Oxygen Consumption

The obvious advantages to quantitating changes in the metabolic rate and, more importantly, the need to compare the metabolic rate to the external respiratory functions require the concept of total body oxygen consumption.

Oxygen consumption refers to the amount of oxygen used by the entire organism in a given time interval.[3] The oxygen content of arterial blood represents the amount of oxygen per 100 ml blood that may *potentially* be delivered to tissues (see Chapter 9). The oxygen content of mixed venous blood (see Chapters 9 and 20) represents the average amount of oxygen remaining in a given volume of blood after tissue extraction of oxygen. The *arterial-mixed venous oxygen content difference* (A-V content difference) represents the average amount of oxygen extracted by the tissues per unit volume of blood. Multiplying the oxygen extracted per unit of blood by the number of units presented to the tissues per minute (cardiac output) allows us to compute the oxygen consumption — expressed in the *Fick equation:*

$$\dot{Q}_T = \frac{\dot{V}_{O_2}}{[Ca_{O_2} - C\bar{v}_{O_2}]}$$

This equation is usually written as:

$$\dot{V}_{O_2} = \dot{Q}_T[Ca_{O_2} - C\bar{v}_{O_2}]$$

$\dot{Q}T$ is total cardiac output (L/min); $\dot{V}_{O_2}$ is oxygen consumed (ml oxygen/min); Ca_{O_2} is oxygen content of arterial blood; $C\bar{v}_{O_2}$ is oxygen content of mixed venous blood (ml oxygen/100 ml blood).

Cardiovascular Physiology

The movement of oxygen from blood to tissue occurs in response to the capillary oxygen tension being greater than the tissue oxygen tension. In general, the greater the gradient, the greater the potential bulk movement of oxygen. *Tissue oxygen tensions* are essentially determined by the rate of utilization of oxygen by the cells; *capillary oxygen tensions* are primarily a function of arterial oxygen contents (see Chapter 9).

The transit time of blood within the capillaries is primarily determined by the cardiovascular system. For convenience and ease of physiologic analysis, the cardiovascular system may be subdivided into three divisions: (1) cor (heart), (2) conduits (vessels), and (3) content (blood).

Cor

The heart is essentially two pumps in a series; the right ventricle pumps blood to the pulmonary circulation (a low-resistance system), and the left ventricle pumps blood to the systemic circulation (a high-resistance system). Under normal circumstances the functions of the right and left ventricles are appropriately matched — ensuring equal outputs by both ventricles. The function of the heart is to supply enough mechanical energy to maintain an adequate flow (perfusion) throughout the vascular system. This flow is expressed as cardiac output ($\dot{Q}$) and is usually given in liters per minute (L/min). The cardiac output is the amount of blood pumped with each beat (stroke volume = SV) times the number of beats per minute (frequency = f):

$$\dot{Q} = SV \times f$$

Cardiac output is directly related to potential oxygen delivery to tissues. An increase in cardiac output allows for less extraction of oxygen per unit volume of blood (assuming a constant metabolic rate). Such an increase in cardiac output represents an important compensatory mechanism for hypoxemia and hypoxia (see Chapter 9).

The slower the blood moves through the capillary, the greater is the degree of oxygen extraction from the blood, assuming that the metabolic rate is constant. This slower rate of movement through the capillary results in a greater arterial to venous oxygen content difference. Since cardiac output plays a major role in determining capillary flow (transit time), it is a major factor in determining the oxygen content of mixed venous blood (see Chapters 9 and 20).

Conduits

This portion of the cardiovascular system includes all of the vessels in the circulation from the large arteries through the microcirculation to the great veins. It may be thought of as having four discreet subdivisions, each with its own function: distribution vessels (aorta, pulmonary artery, large arteries); resistance vessels (arterioles); exchange vessels (metarterioles, thoroughfare channels, true capillaries) — known as the *microcirculation;* and capacitance vessels (venules, great veins, superior and inferior vena cava).

It is essential to remember that there are two major capillary beds: the pulmonary circulation normally containing 30–35% of the circulating blood volume and the systemic circulation normally containing 65–70% of the circulating blood volume. The capacitance (venous) vessels contain the bulk of the blood volume (approximately 65–70%).[8] It is important for the maintenance of adequate perfusion that the capacitance vessels are able to increase or decrease tone.

The systemic vascular system has an important role in the exchange of oxygen between blood and tissues inasmuch as blood must go through the systemic capillaries (microcirculatory system) if it is to supply oxygen to the tissues. The systemic microcirculatory system is somewhat self-regulating, with numerous mechanisms that alter blood flow to the various tissues, including such substances as epinephrine, norepinephrine, histamine, and the many tissue metabolites produced by the cells themselves.

Factors such as tissue pH, Pco_2, and Po_2 play an important role in regulating perfusion. Under normal circumstances the systemic capillary unit dilates and increases blood flow in response to decreased tissue oxygenation (hypoxia), decreased pH, and increased carbon dioxide tensions. Conversely, there will be a degree of vasoconstriction when blood flow to the tissues is excessive.

In some pathophysiologic states the microcirculatory system allows the majority of the blood to go directly from the artery to the vein. This arterial-venous shunting results not only in decreased tissue oxygenation but also in venous oxygen contents above the normal expected value.

Content

The liquid portion of the blood is known as *plasma* and has crucial functions such as coagulation, defense, and maintenance of osmotic relationships. Of course, dissolved oxygen and carbon dioxide exist in the plasma.

The *formed* elements of the blood include red blood cells, white blood cells, and platelets. The percent of the blood volume that is composed of formed elements is known as the *hematocrit*.

If blood is allowed to clot, the remaining liquid portion is called *serum*.

7 / The Physiology of External Respiration

GAS EXCHANGE between blood and the external environment occurs in the pulmonary capillary bed—a process called *external respiration.* The quantities of carbon dioxide and oxygen exchanged must logically equal the exchange in the systemic capillaries, oxygen being added to the blood while carbon dioxide is being removed. This relationship of volumes of carbon dioxide and oxygen exchanged per minute by the lungs is the *respiratory exchange ratio* (RR).[10] The respiratory exchange ratio represents the *overall* exchange capability of the lung, not individual variances occurring within different parts of the lung.[5]

An alternative method of expressing the effectiveness of pulmonary gas exchange is to consider the "matching" of ventilation and perfusion or, more precisely, the relationship between the volume of gas moving into an alveolus and the blood flow through the adjacent capillary.[12] The advantage of this approach is that it takes into account the *efficiency* of molecular gas exchange in all areas of the lung. It is difficult to fully comprehend the complex ventilation to perfusion relationship; however, a basic understanding of the concept is necessary for the clinical application of blood gas measurements.

Distribution of Pulmonary Perfusion

The normal distribution of blood flow throughout the pulmonary vasculature is dependent upon three major factors: (1) gravity, (2) cardiac output, and (3) pulmonary vascular resistance.

Gravity

In normal man standing erect, there is a distance of approximately 30 cm from the *apex* (top) to the *base* (bottom) of the lung. Assuming the pulmonary artery enters the lung halfway between top and bottom, the pulmonary artery pressure would have to be great enough to overcome a gravitational force of 15 cm of water in order to supply flow to the apex; a similar gradient would be aiding flow to the lung base. A column of blood (essentially H_2O) 15 cm high exerts a pressure of approximately 11 mm Hg. *This gravitational effect on blood flow results in a lateral wall pulmonary artery pressure at the lung base of greater magnitude than the pulmonary artery pressure at the*

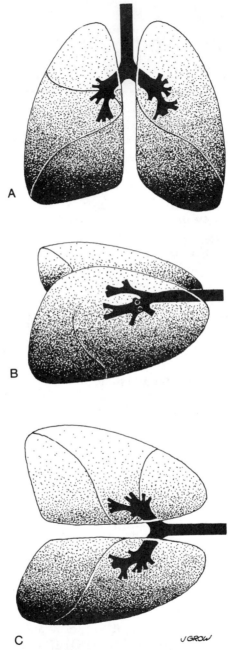

Fig 7–1. — The preponderance of pulmonary blood flow will normally occur in the gravity-dependent areas of the lung. Thus, body position has a significant effect on the distribution of pulmonary blood flow, as shown in the erect **(A),** supine (lying on the back) **(B),** and lateral (lying on the side) **(C)** positions.

apex.[12] Thus, blood will preferentially flow through the gravity-dependent areas of the lung (Fig 7 – 1).

Under normal circumstances, *alveolar* pressures are equal throughout the lung. Theoretically, the least gravity-dependent areas of the lung (the apex in the upright subject) may have alveolar pressures higher than the pulmonary arterial pressures at that level. This would result in the virtual absence of blood flow to these areas. It should be noted that the total absence of pulmonary blood flow to these areas does *not* exist to any significant extent in the normally perfused lung.[77] However, if pulmonary artery pressure is significantly decreased (e.g., shock) or alveolar pressures significantly increased (e.g., intermittent positive-pressure breathing or positive end-expiratory pressure), the absence of perfusion to the least gravity-dependent areas of the lung may become significant.

THE THREE-ZONE MODEL. — It has become well accepted to refer to the gravity effects of pulmonary perfusion in terms of the three-zone model (Fig 7 – 2).[12] Zone 3 is the gravity-dependent area of constant blood flow (arterial pressure greater than alveolar pressure); zone 1 is the least gravity-dependent area of potentially no blood flow (alveolar pressure greater than arterial pressure). The interceding area is zone 2, an area of complex and varying intermittent blood flow.

Fig 7–2. — The three-zone model illustrating the effects of gravity on pulmonary perfusion (see text).

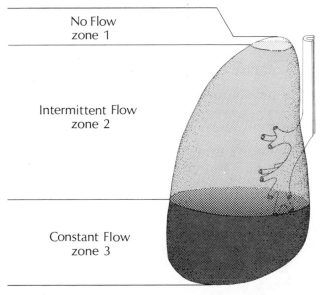

No Flow
zone 1

Intermittent Flow
zone 2

Constant Flow
zone 3

The presence or absence of blood flow in zone 2 depends primarily on the relationship of pulmonary artery pressure to alveolar pressure. Under normal circumstances this is determined far more by the cardiac cycle (systole and diastole) than by the ventilatory cycle (inspiration and expiration).

AUTOREGULATION. — The pulmonary vascular system is a low-pressure system and therefore would be more affected by gravitational forces than would the higher-pressure systemic vascular system. In addition, the systemic vascular system tends to react actively to changes in arterial pressure; that is, the vascular system attempts to actively control the distribution of blood flow in reaction to pressure changes.[3] In contrast, the pulmonary vascular system tends to react passively to changes in pressure, thus accentuating the gravity effect on the distribution of pulmonary perfusion.[78]

Cardiac Output

The amount of blood ejected by the right ventricle per unit time (cardiac output) is a major determinant of blood flow through the pulmonary vasculature. In general, *the greater the cardiac output, the greater the pulmonary artery pressure*. Thus, in the normal lung, as the cardiac output increases, zone 3 extends upward (see Fig 7–2); conversely, as the cardiac output decreases, zone 3 descends. Since the pulmonary vascular system tends to react *passively* to changes in arterial pressure, the gravity effect on the distribution of blood flow secondary to cardiac output changes is greater in the pulmonary system than in the systemic circulation.[12]

Pulmonary Vascular Resistance

Although the pulmonary arterioles are less active in autoregulation than are their systemic counterparts, they are nonetheless capable of causing significant increases in resistance to blood flow.

CHRONIC PULMONARY HYPERTENSION. — This is usually the result of periarteriolar fibrosis within the lung parenchyma.[1] *Chronic pulmonary hypertension* results in increased right ventricular work. Over the long run the right heart meets these increased demands by musculature hypertrophy; that is, the right heart becomes larger. Right ventricular hypertrophy due to chronic pulmonary hypertension is known as *cor pulmonale* — a common problem in patients with chronic lung diseases.

ACUTE PULMONARY HYPERTENSION.—Acute increases in pulmonary vascular resistance will usually result in acute pulmonary hypertension. Of course, acute pulmonary hypertension will result only if the right ventricle is capable of maintaining an adequate cardiac output; if not, the result is right heart failure.

Acute increase in pulmonary vascular resistance is a common phenomenon in critically ill patients. There are three factors that most commonly cause acute increases in pulmonary vascular resistance: (1) decreased alveolar oxygen tensions, (2) acidemia, and (3) arterial hypoxemia.

1. *Decreased alveolar oxygen tension.*—Vasoconstriction occurs in vessels adjacent to alveoli with low oxygen tensions.[79] This local vasoconstriction is believed to play a significant role in diverting blood flow to lung areas where alveolar oxygen tensions are higher.[3]

2. *Acidemia.*—Decreased blood pH tends to produce pulmonary vascular constriction.[5] Acidemia is a common cause of acute pulmonary hypertension and may precipitate right heart failure.

3. *Arterial hypoxemia* (decreased arterial oxygen tension).—Available evidence makes it reasonable to assume that severe hypoxemia may cause reflex-mediated increases in pulmonary vascular resistance.[80]

Certainly, combinations of the above three factors potentiate each other and result in marked pulmonary arteriolar vasoconstriction.

Distribution of Ventilation

Ventilation is the movement of gases in and out of the pulmonary system.[4] To respire, inspired gases must reach the alveolar epithelium. Since all gas is not expelled from the lungs with each expiration, there will be mixing of fresh inspired gases with gases that have previously undergone gas exchange with pulmonary blood flow.[81]

The distribution of inspired gases throughout the pulmonary tree and lung parenchyma is normally dependent upon two major factors: airway resistance and alveolar physics.

Airway Resistance

Gas flows from a region of higher pressure to one of lower pressure. Obviously, the rate at which a volume of gas is displaced (flow) is a function of the pressure gradient and the resistances to that gas flow. Thus, the following statement may be made: resistance equals pressure gradient divided by flow ($R = \Delta P/F$).

LAMINAR FLOW. — *Laminar gas flow* refers to a streamlined molecular flow in which there is little friction between the molecules of gas themselves; there is friction primarily between the molecules and the sides of the tube (Fig 7 – 3). Laminar flow follows the general principle of Poiseuille, which demonstrates that at a constant driving pressure, the flow rate of a gas will vary directly with the fourth power of the radius of the airway. Thus, small changes in airway caliber may greatly affect the delivery of air to the alveoli.

TURBULENT FLOW. — *Turbulent flow* is when gas molecules interreact in a random manner (see Fig 7 – 3). The resistances are not only at the sides of the tube but are also caused by molecular collision of the gases. All other factors being equal, resistance to flow is considerably greater when the flow is turbulent as opposed to laminar.

SMALL AIRWAY DISEASE. — Large airways are normally responsible for 45% of the total airway resistance and, of course, this can be tremendously increased by obstruction caused by such factors as foreign material or swelling of the upper airway.[5] Resistance to gas flow is markedly affected by the patency of individual airways. The large airways (trachea and bronchi) have a significant amount of structural rigidity and are relatively large in diameter, whereas the small airways (bronchioles) are small in diameter and depend in large part on transmural pressure gradients for their patency.[10] In the normal lung, resistances to air flow are equal throughout the pulmonary tree; in

Fig 7–3. — Schematic concept of laminar gas flow **(a)** and turbulent gas flow **(b).** (From Shapiro, B. A., Harrison, R. A., and Trout, C. A.: *Clinical Application of Respiratory Care* [Chicago: Year Book Medical Publishers, Inc., 1975].)

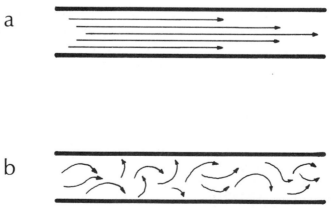

disease states, variances in small airway resistances are a common cause of uneven distribution of ventilation.[82]

Intrathoracic Pressures

Elasticity is the property of matter that causes it to return to its resting state after being deformed by some external force. At the end of a normal expiration there are chest wall elastic forces tending to expand the intrathoracic volume. These forces are balanced by lung tissue elastic forces that tend to reduce the intrathoracic volume (Fig 7–4). The communication linking these two opposing forces is the *pleura;* its visceral layer is attached to the lung and its parietal layer is attached to the chest wall. The visceral and parietal pleurae are held together by a film of fluid in a manner similar to two glass microscope slides that are wet and stuck together. The slides readily move back and forth but resist being pulled apart.

The pleural space is a *potential* space between the two layers of pleura, which is normally occupied by a small amount of fluid. The average resting intrapleural pressure is approximately 4–5 cm of water *less* than the atmospheric pressure. This subatmospheric pressure is a result of the opposing elastic forces of the thorax and lung. The alveoli remain open at the end of expiration because a *distending pressure* exists; that is, alveolar pressures are greater than intrapleural pressure.

Due to factors such as the weight of the lung suspended from the hilum and the gravity distribution of blood flow, the normal resting intrathoracic pressures in the least gravity-dependent portions of the thorax are more negative than the pressures in the more gravity-dependent portion.[12] In erect man (Fig 7–5), assuming alveolar pressures are equal, the alveoli at the apex will be larger because the intrathoracic pressure is more negative; that is, the distending pressure is greater for the apical alveoli than for the basilar alveoli. In essence, then, alveoli are larger in the least gravity-dependent areas of the lung.

Alveolar Physics

This difference in alveolar size is important primarily because an alveolus is essentially a highly elastic semisphere. Since all elastic spheres behave according to the physical *law of Laplace*, this law becomes essential for understanding the effect of alveolar size on the distribution of ventilation.

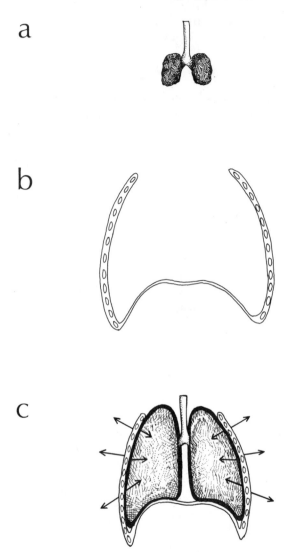

Fig 7–4.—**a** represents resting state of normal lungs when removed from the chest cavity; i.e., elasticity causes total collapse. **b** represents resting state of normal chest wall and diaphragm when apex is open to atmosphere and the thoracic contents removed. **c** represents end expiration in the normal, intact thorax. Note that elastic forces of lung and chest wall are in opposite directions. The pleural surfaces link these two opposing forces (see text). (From Shapiro, B. A., Harrison, R. A., and Trout, C. A.: *Clinical Application of Respiratory Care* [Chicago: Year Book Medical Publishers, Inc., 1975].)

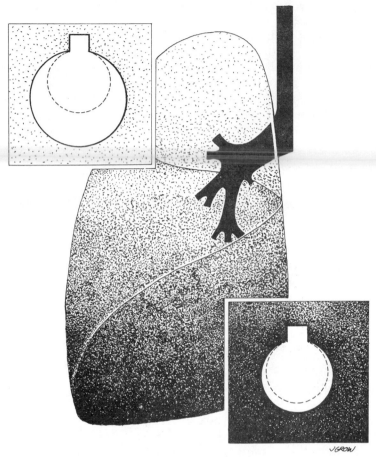

Fig 7–5. — *Dotted circles* represent theoretical critical volumes. Apical alveoli are larger than basilar alveoli in normal erect man because of greater distending pressure in the apical area (see text).

LAW OF LAPLACE. — The Laplace equation, as applied to geometric spheres, states: $P = 2 \times T/R$. P is the distending pressure within the alveolus (dynes/sq cm); T is surface tension of the alveolar fluid (dynes/cm); and R is the radius of the alveolus (cm).

This relationship indicates that the distending pressure necessary to expand the alveolus is determined by (1) the surface tension properties of the liquid substance lining the sphere and (2) the radius of the curvature of the sphere. Inherent in this relationship is the fact that if surface tension remains unchanged, *the smaller the radius, the greater the distending pressure must become to maintain the alveolar volume.*

If such a situation truly existed in the lung, all alveoli would have to be the same size so that the smaller alveoli would not empty their air into the larger ones. However, all alveoli are not the same size; in fact, some alveoli are four to five times larger than others. If surface tension remained constant, the inspiratory air flow would preferentially inflate the larger alveoli, while little or no air entered the smaller alveoli. The result would obviously be one huge, extended alveolus, with all of the others totally collapsed.

SURFACTANT. — The obvious reconciliation of this mechanical dilemma would be to alter the surface tension of the alveolar fluid lining so that a state of equilibrium could be maintained. *Surface tension* is the molecular force present on the surface of a liquid which tends to make the surface area exposed to the atmosphere as small as possible. Simply stated, the molecules on the surface of water are much closer together than they are elsewhere in the fluid. In an elastic sphere, surface tension would play a very major role in the tendency for that sphere to collapse. A substance called pulmonary *surfactant* decreases alveolar surface tension and allows for the appropriate variability to maintain properly functioning alveoli.[83]

ALVEOLAR CRITICAL VOLUME. — All alveoli have a critical volume — a volume below which elastic forces become overwhelming and cause complete collapse of the alveolus.[84] One might think of the critical volume as the alveolar volume below which surface tension constantly exceeds the distending pressure. This causes the radius to become progressively smaller until ultimately the alveolus collapses. Figure 7–5 illustrates the variability of alveolar size and the concept of critical volume.

SUMMARY. — There is a critical volume at which the available distending pressure can equal or exceed the external elastic forces which are tending to collapse the alveolus. Below this critical volume, these external forces are overwhelming and total collapse eventually ensues. Above the critical volume, the surface acting substances work in such a way as to maintain a dynamic state of equilibrium. This is accomplished by a balance between the distending pressures tending to inflate the alveolus (alveolar pressure minus intrapleural pressure) and the surface tension properties tending to collapse the alveolus.

The following generalization concerning the behavior of alveoli that remain above their critical volume may be made: Small alveoli resist expansion but contract rapidly (fast alveoli); large alveoli expand readily (until a maximum volume is reached) but contract slowly (slow alveoli). These factors have profound effects on the distribution of ventilation not only in the normal lung but also in numerous disease states.

Ventilation to Perfusion Relationship

Gravity distribution of perfusion causes differences in perfusion pressures at various levels of the lung. In an erect man, at the lung bases the lateral wall pulmonary artery pressures are much higher than at the apices. Differences in intrapleural pressures result in the alveoli being smaller at the bases and larger at the apices.

At normal lung volumes, the greater portion of the tidal volume goes to the bases largely because of alveolar size differentials. In other words, small alveoli have larger volume changes per unit time than do the larger alveoli.[81] The net result is that under normal conditions most of the air exchange takes place at the bases in coincidence with most of the blood flow. *Thus, in the normal lung most of the total ventilation and even more of the total blood flow go to the gravity-dependent areas.*[12]

Of all the physiologic alterations resulting from various pulmonary diseases, the problem of uneven distribution of ventilation is the most common and crucial. Any disease that causes changes in the elastic properties of the alveoli or causes pulmonary mucosal edema, inflammation, plugging of the bronchioles, or bronchospasm may result in uneven air distribution to alveoli.

Shunting and Deadspace

The basic pulmonary gas exchange unit is a single alveolus with its associated pulmonary capillary. This theoretical respiratory unit can exist in one of four relationships (Fig 7–6): (1) the *normal unit* is one in which ventilation and perfusion are relatively equal; (2) a *deadspace unit* is one in which the alveolus is normally ventilated but there is no blood flow through the capillary—the alveolar gas cannot participate in molecular blood-gas exchange; (3) in a *shunt unit* the alveolus is completely unventilated while the adjacent capillary has blood flow—the blood goes from the right heart to the left heart without undergoing gas exchange; (4) a *silent unit* is one in which both the alveolus and the capillary are completely collapsed.

Any one of these absolute conditions may exist in the lungs at any time. An infinite number of ventilation-perfusion relationships may

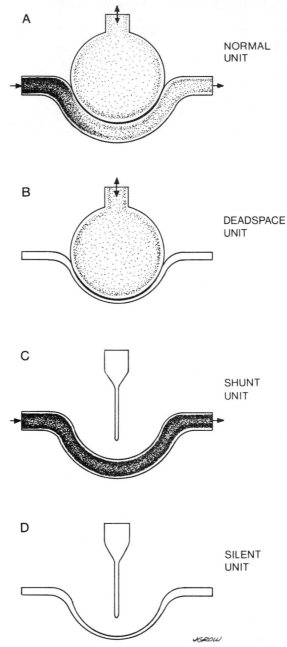

Fig 7–6.—The theoretical respiratory unit. **A,** normal ventilation, normal perfusion; **B,** normal ventilation, no perfusion; **C,** no ventilation, normal perfusion; **D,** no ventilation, no perfusion.

exist between the deadspace unit, the normal unit, and the shunt unit. This spectrum is illustrated in Figure 7–7. The complexities of the ventilation-perfusion ratio are primarily due to the spectrum between the two extremes of deadspace and shunt.

Fig 7–7.—The spectrum of ventilation to perfusion relationships. As shown, *a* represents the spectrum of ventilation in excess of perfusion; *b* represents the spectrum of perfusion in excess of ventilation. The true deadspace unit is represented as infinite $\dot{V}_A/\dot{Q}$; the normal unit is represented as $\dot{V}_A/\dot{Q}$, equalling one; the shunt unit is represented as zero $\dot{V}_A/\dot{Q}$. (From Shapiro, B. A., Harrison, R. A., and Trout, C. A.: *Clinical Application of Respiratory Care* [Chicago: Year Book Medical Publishers, Inc., 1975].)

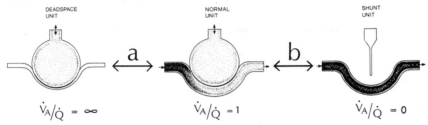

DEADSPACE UNIT   NORMAL UNIT   SHUNT UNIT

$$\dot{V}_A/\dot{Q} = \infty \qquad \dot{V}_A/\dot{Q} = 1 \qquad \dot{V}_A/\dot{Q} = 0$$

8 / Arterial Carbon Dioxide Tension

THE MOST physiologically reflective blood gas measurement is the arterial carbon dioxide tension (Pa_{CO_2}). It directly reflects the adequacy of alveolar ventilation; i.e., it tells how well air is exchanging with blood in the lungs. Only when the factors determining Pa_{CO_2} are thoroughly understood can the full meaning of this measurement be appreciated.

The means by which the blood carries carbon dioxide (CO_2 transport) is highly complex (see Chapter 3). As a review, three generalizations may be stated:

1.   Almost all (approximately 95%) of the carbon dioxide in the blood is transported through buffering mechanisms present in the red blood cell. A very small portion actually is dissolved in the plasma (see Fig 3–3).

2.   The *dissolved* carbon dioxide determines the blood partial pressure, thus it is the only blood factor that participates in determining the carbon dioxide pressure gradient with alveolar air or tissue. This pressure gradient plays a major role in determining whether carbon dioxide enters or leaves the blood and at what rate it does so. In other words, *the dissolved carbon dioxide determines the blood portion of the pressure gradient.*

3.   The quantity of carbon dioxide the blood is capable of accepting or giving up depends to a great extent on the buffering systems (see Chapter 3). In most circumstances this natural blood-buffering capability is not exceeded, and therefore the carbon dioxide tension is the only significant determinant of the extent to which the blood accepts or gives up carbon dioxide. We will always assume this to be the case.

Carbon Dioxide Homeostasis

If one removes from the cardiopulmonary homeostatic schema (see Fig 5–1) all of the factors that do not affect the moment-to-moment control of the arterial carbon dioxide tension, there remains an exquisitely simple relationship (Fig 8–1): *The metabolic rate of the body is balanced against the effectiveness of ventilation.* On the one hand, the metabolic rate determines the rate and amount of carbon dioxide that enters the venous blood; on the other, the effective ventilation determines the alveolar carbon dioxide tension and, therefore, how much carbon dioxide will be excreted in the lung.

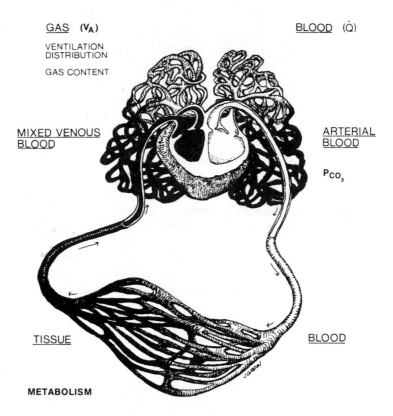

EXTERNAL RESPIRATION

Fig 8–1.—The carbon dioxide homeostatic schema. This schema is the result of removing all factors in the cardiopulmonary homeostatic schema (see Fig 5–1) that do not affect carbon dioxide homeostasis. The arterial P_{CO_2} is determined by the relationship between tissue metabolism and alveolar ventilation.

Total Ventilation

Ventilation is the mass movement of gases into and out of the pulmonary system.[4] This *total ventilation* is clinically measured by *pulmonary function studies.* As depicted in Figure 8–2, *total lung ca-*

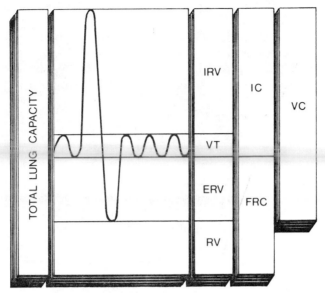

Fig 8–2. — The divisions of total lung capacity. Total lung capacity (TLC) is the maximum amount of air the lungs can hold. The total lung capacity is divided into four primary volumes: inspiratory reserve volume (IRV), tidal volume (VT), expiratory reserve volume (ERV), and residual volume (RV). Assuming a normal male with TLC of 6,000 ml: IRV = 3,100 ml, VT = 500 ml, ERV = 1,200 ml, and RV = 1,200 ml.

Capacities are combinations of two or more lung volumes. They are inspiratory capacity (IC), functional residual capacity (FRC), and vital capacity (VC).

pacity (TLC) is defined as the maximum amount of air the lungs can hold. It is divided into four *primary* volumes.

1. *Tidal volume* (VT) — the amount of air moved into or out of the lungs. Resting tidal volume is the normal volume of air inhaled or exhaled in one breath.

2. *Inspiratory reserve volume* (IRV) — the amount of air that can be forcefully inspired after a normal tidal volume inhalation.

3. *Expiratory reserve volume* (ERV) — the amount of air that can be forcefully exhaled after a normal tidal volume exhalation.

4. *Residual volume* (RV) — the amount of air left in the lungs after a forced exhalation.

Capacities are combinations of volumes:

1. *Vital capacity* (VC) = IRV + VT + ERV. This is the amount of air that can be forcefully exhaled after a maximal inspiration.

    a. *Slow vital capacity* (SVC) is the VC when no effort is made to exhale rapidly.

    b. *Forced vital capacity* (FVC) is the VC when a maximal effort is made to exhale as rapidly as possible. If the FVC is timed, it is possible to measure *forced expiratory volume per unit time,* such as FEV_1 (forced expiratory volume in 1 second).

2. *Inspiratory capacity* (IC) = V_T + IRV.

3. *Functional residual capacity* (FRC) = ERV + RV. It is measured by a method involving inert gas (helium or nitrogen) equilibration.

4. *Total lung capacity* (TLC) = IC + FRC.

The most common clinical measurement of total ventilation in respiratory care is either tidal volume (V_T) or minute volume (MV).[11] The minute volume is the product of the tidal volume and the respiratory rate (RR).

Effective and Wasted Ventilation

In the living organism a portion of the total ventilation respires, i.e., undergoes molecular gas exchange with pulmonary blood. Thus, the total ventilation per unit time is composed of gas that respires (alveolar ventilation) and gas that does not respire (deadspace ventilation):

$$\dot{V} = \dot{V}_A + \dot{V}_D$$

Alveolar Ventilation ($\dot{V}_A$)

In general, only the portion of total ventilation that respires has positive physiologic significance; that is, it is the physiologically effective portion of the total ventilation. This *effective ventilation* is most commonly referred to as *alveolar ventilation — that portion of the total ventilation that undergoes molecular gas exchange with pulmonary blood.*[2]

Deadspace Ventilation ($\dot{V}_D$)

The portion of the total ventilation that does *not* respire is wasted ventilation, i.e., *not* physiologically effective. This wasted ventilation is most commonly called *deadspace ventilation — that portion of the total ventilation that does NOT undergo molecular gas exchange with pulmonary blood.*[2]

Deadspace ventilation may result from one of three circumstances:

1.   Anatomic deadspace. — *The volume of air contained in the pulmonary conducting system* is the anatomic deadspace. In spontaneous breathing the volume of the conducting system is fairly constant; and this is to say that the volume of the conducting system is consistently related to normal body size. *The anatomic deadspace is usually equal to 1 ml/pound (2.2 ml/kg) of normal body weight.*

2.   Alveolar deadspace. — If an alveolus is being ventilated but the pulmonary capillary is not being perfused, the air in that alveolus is deadspace ventilation, i.e., the air is not exchanging with pulmonary blood (see Fig 7–6). Unlike anatomic deadspace, alveolar deadspace can be highly variable and unpredictable.

3.   Deadspace effect. — When ventilation in excess of perfusion exists, two results are theoretically possible. The greater air exchange in the alveolus may result in better alveolar ventilation; i.e., there is decreased PA_{co_2} and Pa_{co_2}. However, part or all of the increased alveolar air exchange may *not* respire. Such a ventilation/perfusion inequality may be due either to overventilation or to underperfusion. This is the component of deadspace ventilation that responds most markedly to changes in total ventilation or total pulmonary blood flow.

Ventilatory Pattern

Every tidal volume includes anatomic deadspace. The larger the tidal volume, the less significant the anatomic deadspace. The more rapid the respiratory rate, the greater the portion of the minute ventilation that will be anatomic deadspace. Figure 8–3 demonstrates how, in spite of a constant minute volume, changes in ventilatory pattern alter the alveolar, or effective, ventilation. When we add to this information the fact that total deadspace ventilation varies greatly with disease, it becomes obvious that *clinical observations of ventilation may be totally inadequate for assessing the physiologic adequacy of ventilation.*

Arterial Carbon Dioxide Tension (Pa_{CO_2})

The metabolic rate is a major determinant of tissue carbon dioxide tension. This means that the arterial-venous carbon dioxide tension difference is primarily determined by the metabolic rate. The metabolic rate, therefore, is an important factor in determining the mixed venous (pulmonary artery) carbon dioxide tension ($P\bar{v}_{co_2}$).

The movement of carbon dioxide from pulmonary blood to alveolar

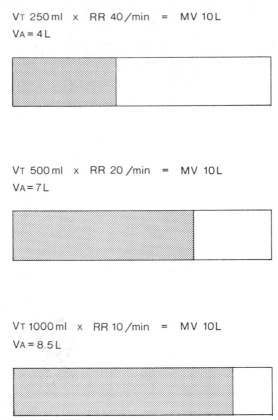

Fig 8–3.—The ventilatory pattern and alveolar ventilation. In all three examples the minute volume (MV) is 10 L. Assuming an anatomic deadspace of 150 ml, the alveolar ventilation (VA) varies markedly with changes in ventilatory pattern (VT = tidal volume; RR = respiratory rate). Obviously, disease can add deadspaces other than the anatomic ones and can cause even greater variances in alveolar ventilation.

air is dependent upon the carbon dioxide pressure gradient between pulmonary blood and alveolus. Because carbon dioxide readily diffuses across the alveolar-capillary membrane, we may assume the carbon dioxide tensions are equal in alveolar air and arterial blood.[9] This is shown schematically in Figure 8–4.

Arterial carbon dioxide tension (Pa_{CO_2}) is a direct reflection of how well the lungs are exchanging air with blood in relation to the metabolic rate. In other words, *the Pa_{CO_2} is the direct and immediate reflection of the adequacy of alveolar ventilation in relation to the metabolic rate.*

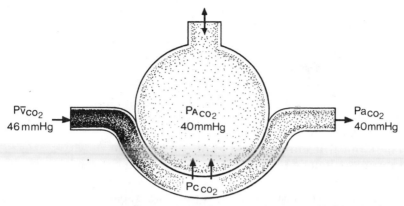

Fig 8–4. — Major factors determining alveolar carbon dioxide tension. Inspired air normally is void of a significant carbon dioxide tension; therefore alveolar carbon dioxide tension (PA_{CO_2}) must be the net result of fresh air exchange in the alveolus in relation to mixed venous carbon dioxide tension ($P\bar{v}_{CO_2}$). Carbon dioxide diffusion is normally so rapid that total equilibrium must occur between pulmonary capillary carbon dioxide tension (Pc_{CO_2}) and PA_{CO_2}. This means that arterial carbon dioxide tension (Pa_{CO_2}) should equal PA_{CO_2}. Normal values are illustrated.

To emphasize the clinical importance of the arterial carbon dioxide tension measurement, remember that the physiologic criterion of adequate lung function is how well the metabolic demands of the body are being met. The assessment of adequate physiologic ventilation is accomplished through arterial carbon dioxide tension measurement. Differentiation and classification of pulmonary diseases are accomplished by pulmonary function studies and other methods, *but the physiologic assessment of the adequacy of ventilation is by Pa_{CO_2} measurement.*

Quantitating the Deadspace

The Pa_{CO_2} measurement clinically quantitates the effectiveness of alveolar ventilation in relation to metabolism. It would be desirable to quantitate deadspace ventilation so easily. Unfortunately, such a measurement does not exist, thus requiring less satisfactory and more complicated methods to be used.

There are circumstances in which it would seem quite apparent that abnormal increases in deadspace exist. A good example is the clinical observation of a patient breathing three to four times his normal predicted minute volume and yet having a normal arterial carbon dioxide tension. This patient's increase in deadspace ventilation must be significant since there has been a very large increase in total ventilation without any increase in alveolar ventilation (see Chapter 12). In clinical medicine, the presence of increased deadspace is usually not nearly as obvious as in the above example, and a measurement documenting the increase would be clinically helpful. Such a measurement is commonly referred to as the *deadspace to tidal volume ratio* (V_D/V_T) and may be defined as that portion of the tidal volume that does not exchange with pulmonary capillary blood.[2]

The clinical usefulness and application of the deadspace to tidal volume ratio depend upon four factors that must be carefully noted.

1. Both anatomic and alveolar deadspace are being measured, thus it is important to observe that the patient has a reasonably normal ventilatory pattern. This observation rules out significant increases in deadspace ventilation due solely to increases in anatomic deadspace.

2. The metabolic rate must be within normal limits to the extent determinable by clinical observation, i.e., normal temperature, normal muscle activity, etc.

3. Cardiovascular function must be reasonably adequate to reflect the patient's total body tissue production of carbon dioxide.

4. The technical procedures for measuring deadspace to tidal volume ratios must be extremely exact; that is, the entire expired air sample must be collected and care must be taken to prevent any intermittent leak from the expired volume. In the spontaneously breathing patient, a long enough period of time must be allowed for the tidal volume variability to no longer affect the mean expired carbon dioxide tension. This time and variability factor makes the measurement far more practical and accurate for patients controlled on positive-pressure volume ventilators than for spontaneously breathing patients. The values of deadspace to tidal volume ratios in normal spontaneously breathing patients range from 0.2 to 0.4 (20–40%).[2]

Development of the V_D/V_T

The basic premise for quantitating the deadspace to tidal volume ratio is that the total gas volume expired is equal to the sum of the alveolar volume expired and the deadspace volume expired:

$$\dot{V}_E = \dot{V}_A = \dot{V}_D \tag{1}$$

$\dot{V}_E$ is the total gas volume expired; $\dot{V}_A$ is the alveolar gas volume expired; and $\dot{V}_D$ is the deadspace volume expired.

A fraction of the expired gas is carbon dioxide. Over a period of time, the collected CO_2 mixes uniformly within the total expired gas. Comparing the volume of CO_2 collected to the total gas volume collected is expressed as the mean expired fraction of carbon dioxide ($F\bar{E}CO_2$):

$$F\bar{E}CO_2 = \frac{CO_2 \text{ volume collected}}{\text{total volume collected}} \tag{2}$$

The carbon dioxide expired must come from either alveolar or deadspace volume:

$$\dot{V}E \times F\bar{E}CO_2 = (\dot{V}A \times FACO_2) + (\dot{V}D \times FDCO_2) \tag{3}$$

However, the fraction of carbon dioxide in deadspace air approaches that of inspired air (essentially zero). Therefore, equation (3) may be expressed as:

$$\dot{V}E \times F\bar{E}CO_2 = \dot{V}A \times FACO_2 \tag{4}$$

The volume of alveolar ventilation must be equal to the total expired volume minus the deadspace volume:

$$\dot{V}A = (\dot{V}E - \dot{V}D) \tag{5}$$

Inserting this equivalent term for alveolar ventilation into equation (4), multiplying out, and collecting all similar volume terms on each side of the equation result in the following mathematical relationships:

$$\dot{V}E \times F\bar{E}CO_2 = (\dot{V}E - \dot{V}D)FACO_2 \tag{6}$$

$$\dot{V}D \times FACO_2 = \dot{V}E \times FACO_2 - \dot{V}E \times F\bar{E}CO_2 \tag{7}$$

Dividing both sides of equation (7) by the fraction of alveolar carbon dioxide ($FACO_2$) and by the volume expired ($\dot{V}E$) gives:

$$\frac{\dot{V}D}{\dot{V}E} = \frac{FACO_2 - F\bar{E}CO_2}{FACO_2} \tag{8}$$

Two basic relationships are now used to further simplify the equation: (1) the fraction of a gas (FCO_2) is proportional to the partial pressure of the gas (PCO_2); and (2) the alveolar carbon dioxide tensions can be very closely approximated by arterial carbon dioxide tension measurement. The term expired volume ($\dot{V}E$) is used interchangeably with the term tidal volume ($\dot{V}T$). Incorporating these basic relationships into equation (8) gives the *clinical deadspace equation:*

$$\frac{\dot{V}D}{\dot{V}T} = \frac{Pa_{CO_2} - P\bar{E}_{CO_2}}{Pa_{CO_2}} \tag{9}$$

Equation (9) is the form most commonly used to measure dead-space to tidal volume ratios. In a simplified concept it can be visualized that the degree of dilution of alveolar carbon dioxide tension in expired air will increase as the size of the deadspace increases. In other words, the greater the portion of the tidal volume that is deadspace, the less will be the partial pressure of carbon dioxide in the expired air.

9 / Arterial Oxygenation

IN CHAPTER 8 the complexity of cardiopulmonary homeostasis was compared with the simplicity of carbon dioxide homeostasis. Figure 9-1 represents the oxygen homeostatic schema, which is conveyed by removing from the cardiopulmonary schema (see Fig 5-1) the only factors that do not *directly* affect oxygen homeostasis, namely, arterial, mixed venous, and tissue carbon dioxide tension.

Two generalizations should be obvious: (1) the process of ventilation may be conceptually separated from the process of tissue oxygenation and (2) tissue oxygenation involves many factors other than ventilation. In other words, *the biologic processes of oxygenation and ventilation are separate entities.* When evaluating the critically ill patient, it is essential to remember that even though oxygenation and ventilation are separate entities, they are closely interrelated. Poor ventilation may cause inadequate tissue oxygenation (hypoxia); however, tissue oxygenation is often adequate in spite of poor ventilation. On the other hand, adequate ventilation does not insure adequate tissue oxygenation. In summary, *tissue hypoxia may exist when lung function is normal, and tissue oxygenation may be adequate when lung function is very poor.*

Hypoxia is the condition of cellular oxygen deficiency (see Chapter 6). Intracellular measurement of PO_2 is not clinically available at present; however, even if such measurements were available, where would the measurements be made? Vital organs (e.g., heart, brain, and kidney) are not readily available for testing. Skin or skeletal muscles are available tissues but do not always reflect vital organ tissue oxygenation. Therefore, *the diagnosis of hypoxia will remain a clinical judgment in the foreseeable future!*

The measurement of the oxygenation status of the arterial blood provides the clinician with information that can be used in the clinical evaluation of the tissue oxygenation status. Table 6-1 and Figure 9-1 demonstrate that arterial oxygenation is but a factor in the process of tissue oxygenation—however, a factor that can be readily measured.

Defining Hypoxemia

Hypoxemia is traditionally defined as "a relative deficiency of oxygen in the blood";[2, 5, 7, 8] in other words, a state of oxygenation in the

EXTERNAL RESPIRATION

PULMONARY CAPILLARY BED

GAS (V̇A)

VENTILATION
DISTRIBUTION
DIFFUSION
GAS CONTENT

BLOOD (Q̇)

DISTRIBUTION
SHUNTING
CARDIAC OUTPUT

MIXED VENOUS
BLOOD

pH

P_{O_2}
S_{O_2}
Hb
P_{50}

ARTERIAL
BLOOD

pH

P_{O_2}
S_{O_2}
Hb
P_{50}

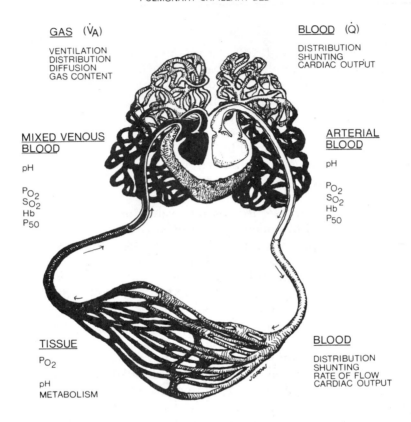

TISSUE

P_{O_2}

pH
METABOLISM

BLOOD

DISTRIBUTION
SHUNTING
RATE OF FLOW
CARDIAC OUTPUT

SYSTEMIC CAPILLARY BED

INTERNAL RESPIRATION

Fig 9–1.—The oxygen homeostatic schema. This schema is the result of removing all factors in the cardiopulmonary homeostatic schema (see Fig 5–1) not directly related to oxygen homeostasis. The only factors removed are those directly concerned with carbon dioxide homeostasis; namely, arterial, mixed venous, and tissue Pco_2.

arterial blood that is less than normal. The Clark electrode (see Chapter 4) has permitted rapid and accurate measurement of the arterial oxygen tension (Pa_{O_2}), as have modern spectrophotometric techniques (see Chapter 4) made oxyhemoglobin measurements available. Over the past twenty years, the Pa_{O_2} measurement has become the primary tool for the clinical evaluation of the arterial oxygenation status.[1, 5, 7, 8, 10, 13]

Keeping in mind that arterial oxygenation involves more than the oxygen tension, this text defines hypoxemia as *a relative deficiency of oxygen tension in the arterial blood.* Such a definition is completely compatible with the current medical literature and lends itself most readily to the clinical care of acutely ill patients.

Thus, hypoxemia denotes that the arterial oxygen tension is below an acceptable range (see Chapter 12). Hypoxemia does not necessarily mean that tissues are hypoxic. It is possible to have normal tissue oxygenation in conjunction with hypoxemia, just as it is possible to have normal arterial oxygen tensions and still have tissue hypoxia. The clinical application of the Pa_{O_2} measurement is primarily based on the concept of arterial blood oxygenation.

Hemoglobin Dissociation Curve

The chemistry of the hemoglobin molecule has been discussed at length (see Chapter 3). The normal range of hemoglobin in the adult is

Fig 9–2. —Hemoglobin and oxygen. Iron sites on the hemoglobin molecule attract oxygen molecules. Oxygen molecules in the alveolus *(upper right)* cross the alveolar-capillary membrane and enter the plasma as dissolved oxygen. The hemoglobin acts as a magnet, and most of the oxygen is removed from solution by attaching to the hemoglobin.

HEMOGLOBIN ◀━━━━━━━━━━━━━ OXYGEN

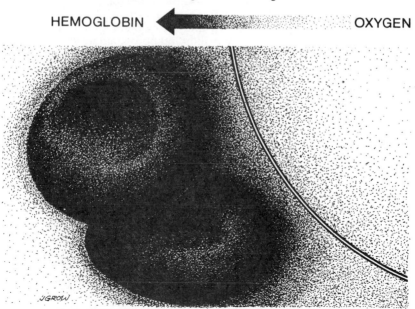

12 – 16 gm/100 ml blood — expressed as grams percent (gm%).[13] Under normal conditions hemoglobin exists primarily in two forms: oxyhemoglobin (HbO_2) and reduced hemoglobin (Hb).

Exposing a solution such as blood to a given partial pressure of oxygen results in oxygen molecules moving into the blood (see Henry's law in Chapter 1). Most of the oxygen entering attaches immediately to the hemoglobin molecule (Fig 9 – 2). Oxygen continues to move from the alveoli into the blood until a pressure gradient between the alveoli and the pulmonary capillary blood no longer exists. At this equilibrium point the hemoglobin is maximally saturated for that blood oxygen tension.

Exposing the hemoglobin to increasing oxygen tensions results in increasing oxyhemoglobin saturation until eventually all the hemoglobin is saturated with oxygen. A sigmoid curve results at oxygen tensions between 0 and 150 mm Hg; this curve is characterized as the *hemoglobin dissociation curve* (Fig 9 – 3). For oxygen tensions between 20 and 80 mm Hg, large amounts of oxygen may be carried and released by the blood with relatively small changes in blood oxygen tensions.

Fig 9–3. — The hemoglobin dissociation curve. This curve shows the relationship of plasma oxygen partial pressure to the degree to which potential oxygen-carrying hemoglobin sites have oxygen attached (% saturation oxygen). This nonlinear relationship accounts for most of the oxygen reserves in blood. Normally, hemoglobin is 50% saturated at a plasma Po_2 of approximately 27 mm Hg; this is designated P_{50}. Normal venous blood has an oxygen partial pressure ($P\bar{v}_{O_2}$) of 40 mm Hg and an oxyhemoglobin saturation of 75%. A Po_2 of 60 mm Hg normally results in approximately 90% saturation. Normal arterial blood has an oxygen partial pressure (Pa_{O_2}) of 97 mm Hg and an oxyhemoglobin saturation of 97%.

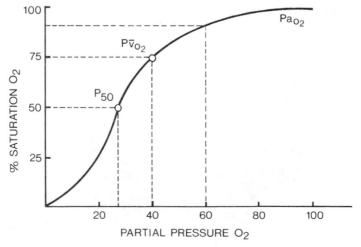

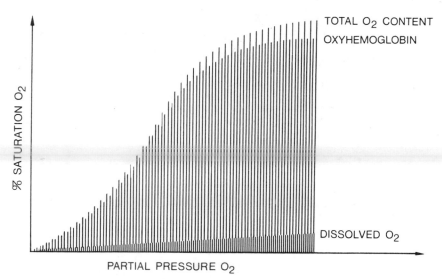

Fig 9–4.—Oxygen content and hemoglobin saturation. Total oxygen content is shown, along with the portion attached to hemoglobin and the portion dissolved in plasma. As long as the hemoglobin is not fully saturated, great increases in oxygen content are seen with small increases in Po_2. In this range almost all of the increase in oxygen content is due to oxygen attached to hemoglobin. When hemoglobin is maximally saturated, large increases in Po_2 are accompanied by small increases in oxygen content, because only increases in dissolved oxygen are possible.

To summarize, the partial pressure of oxygen is critical since it determines the pressure gradient between systemic capillary blood and tissue (as well as between pulmonary capillary blood and alveoli). The quantity of oxygen that may move into (or out of) the blood is dependent upon two factors: the amount of dissolved oxygen and the amount of oxygen that is carried by the hemoglobin. Under normal conditions the quantity of dissolved oxygen is relatively small compared to the total oxygen carried by the blood (Fig 9–4).

Conditions may exist where partial pressures of oxygen are increased up to one atmosphere or more (e.g., high concentrations of inspired oxygen or hyperbaric conditions). In such cases, a metabolically significant amount of oxygen may be carried in the dissolved state. It is essential to make the distinction between oxygen *tension* and oxygen *content*.

Oxygen Content

The traditional studies determined that 1 gm of hemoglobin fully saturated with oxygen could carry 1.34 ml oxygen.[4] These measure-

TABLE 9-1.—CALCULATING OXYGEN CONTENT

Grams percent (gm%) = grams of hemoglobin per 100 ml blood
Volumes percent (vol%) = milliliters of oxygen per 100 ml blood

STEPS
1. Hemoglobin content (gm%) $\times$ 1.34° $\times$ So_2 = oxygen attached to hemoglobin (vol%)
2. Po_2 $\times$ 0.003° = oxygen dissolved in plasma (vol%)
3. Steps 1 + 2 = *oxygen content* (vol%)

Example 1: Hb 15 gm%, Po_2 100 mm Hg, So_2 100%
  1. 15 $\times$ 1.34 $\times$ 1.00 = 20.10 vol%
  2. 100 $\times$ 0.003 = 0.30 vol%

  3.   20.40 vol%

Example 2: Hb 15 gm%, Po_2 50 mm Hg, So_2 85%
  1. 15 $\times$ 1.34 $\times$ 0.85 = 17.09 vol%
  2. 50 $\times$ 0.003   = 0.15 vol%

  3.   17.24 vol%

°For the derivation of these constants see text.

ments involve techniques in which the red blood cells remained intact. Recent work with hemolyzed blood has suggested that a value of approximately 1.39 ml of oxygen may be more representative.[8] Throughout this text the traditional value of 1.34 ml of oxygen will be used.

The quantity of *dissolved* oxygen that may be carried by the blood can be obtained from the Bunsen solubility coefficient for oxygen and blood. For each 100 ml of blood at BTSP,° 0.003 ml of oxygen can be dissolved for each 1 mm Hg of oxygen tension.[4, 8] Thus, 100 ml of blood with an oxygen tension of 100 mm Hg contains 0.3 ml of dissolved oxygen. Milliliters of oxygen dissolved per 100 ml blood are expressed as volumes percent (vol%).

The oxygen content represents the sum of the oxygen attached to hemoglobin and that dissolved in plasma. Thus, blood at BTPS with 15 gm of hemoglobin and 100% saturation has an oxygen content of 20.4 vol%. Steps in the calculation of oxygen content are illustrated in Table 9-1.

Oxygen Affinity

Hemoglobin has a strong affinity for oxygen (see Chapter 3). It is this property of hemoglobin that allows poorly oxygenated blood to oxygenate readily in the pulmonary capillary bed. On the other hand, this affinity for oxygen may make the hemoglobin less able to release

———
°Body temperature, atmospheric pressure, fully saturated with water vapor (see Chapter 1).

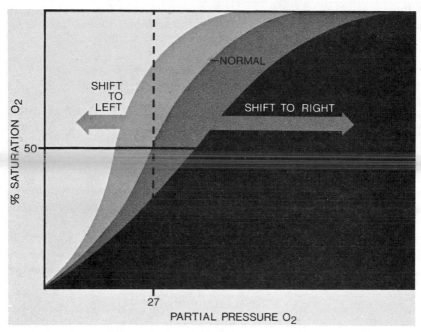

Fig 9–5. — Hemoglobin affinity for oxygen. Increased oxygen affinity *(shift to the left)* means there will be a higher oxygen content at any given Po_2. Conversely, decreased oxygen affinity *(shift to the right)* means there will be a lower oxygen content at any given Po_2. A shift to the left is the result of alkalemia (decreased H^+), hypothermia (cold), hypocarbia (decreased Pco_2), and decreased 2,3-diphosphoglycerate. A shift to the right is the result of acidemia (increased H^+), hyperthermia (fever), hypercarbia (increased Pco_2), and increased 2,3-DPG.

oxygen at the tissue level. Certain factors in the blood alter the affinity and, in so doing, change the normal relationship between hemoglobin saturation and oxygen tension (Fig 9 – 5). In other words, a change in the hemoglobin affinity for oxygen changes the position of the hemoglobin dissociation curve.

Decreased Oxygen Affinity

This is most often referred to as a *shift of the oxygen dissociation curve to the right*. In other words, for any given oxygen tension, there is decreased oxyhemoglobin relative to the normal state. Therefore, for any given oxygen tension, the oxygen transport capability of the blood is decreased because the oxygen content is decreased. A shift to the right aids oxygen movement from blood to tissue in the peripheral capillaries. However, an *extreme* shift to the right almost always results in a decreased oxygen content, which limits the amount of oxygen that may be given to the tissue regardless of how easily it can dissociate from the hemoglobin.

Increased Oxygen Affinity

This is most commonly referred to as a *shift of the dissociation curve to the left*. In other words, for any given oxygen tension, there is increased oxyhemoglobin saturation. It should be obvious that at any given oxygen tension, the oxygen transport capability of the blood is increased since there is increased oxyhemoglobin present. The tissue oxygenation significance of an increased hemoglobin affinity is *potentially* profound. Hemoglobin may be thought of as an oxygen magnet in the blood — the stronger the magnet, the less effective is any given blood to tissue tension gradient for transferring oxygen to the tissues. In other words, the greater the hemoglobin affinity for oxygen, the less potential effectiveness any arterial oxygen tension has in delivering oxygen to the tissues.

Clinical Significance

Physiologic factors such as changes in hydrogen ion concentration, carbon dioxide tension, and temperature affect hemoglobin affinity for oxygen (see Chapter 3).[85] An increase in any of these factors produces a shift of the oxygen dissociation curve to the right (see Fig 9–5). Conversely, a decrease in any of these factors produces a shift to the left. Under normal circumstances these factors work to the physiologic benefit of the organism. For example, tissue metabolism produces hydrogen ions and carbon dioxide, which result in a slight shift of the oxygen dissociation curve to the right and a slight decrease in the affinity of hemoglobin for oxygen. This process results in increased amounts of oxygen available for transfer to the tissues. However, in disease states these relationships may not benefit the organism. For example, when there is a sudden *severe* shift to the right, there is a resultant decrease in oxygen available for the tissues. Thus, sudden and severe acidemia and/or hypercarbia cause decreased oxygen content and, therefore, potentially decreased oxygen availability to the tissues.

P_{50}

Studies of red blood cells have revealed that certain enzyme systems are responsible for aiding the dissociation of oxygen from hemoglobin (see Chapter 3). Many phosphorylase enzyme systems seem to be involved, but the most completely studied at present is the enzyme producing the substrate 2,3-diphosphoglycerate (2,3-DPG). This enzyme system enhances the dissociation of oxygen from hemoglobin by competing with oxygen for the iron-binding site.[86] Thus, lowered levels of the enzyme will produce an increased hemoglobin affinity for oxygen, which has the same effect as shifting the curve to the left. The laboratory ability to measure such changes led to the development of the P_{50} measurement.

The P_{50} is defined as the oxygen tension at which 50% of the hemoglobin is saturated under very specific conditions of laboratory measurement: 37°C, P_{CO_2} 40 mm Hg, and pH 7.40.[87, 88] Figure 9–6 illustrates the concept of the P_{50} measurement. Whatever the laboratory method for determining P_{50}, the conditions of a pH of 7.40, a P_{CO_2} of 40 mm Hg, and a body temperature of 37°C must be included. In most laboratories P_{CO_2} and pH are calculated in the final determination.[89] It must be emphasized that pH, P_{CO_2}, and temperature changes in the patient will affect the hemoglobin affinity for oxygen (see Fig 9–5) but will not affect the P_{50} measurement.

The normal adult P_{50} is approximately 27 mm Hg; in other words, normal adult hemoglobin is 50% saturated at a P_{O_2} of 27 mm Hg when the temperature is 37°C, the P_{CO_2} is 40 mm Hg, and the pH is 7.40.[90] A

Fig 9–6. — P_{50}, a measurement of oxygen affinity. At normal pH and temperature the hemoglobin curve will be such that 50% of the hemoglobin will be saturated at a P_{O_2} of 27–28 mm Hg. If hemoglobin affinity for oxygen is increased for some reason other than alkalemia, cold, or hypocapnia, hemoglobin will be 50% saturated at a lower P_{O_2}. Thus, a P_{50} of 20 mm Hg means the oxygen affinity is increased.

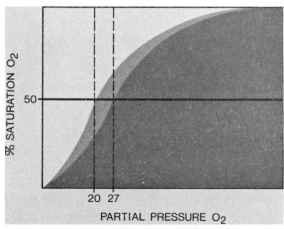

reduced P_{50} means an increased hemoglobin affinity for oxygen. This phenomenon has been studied in stored blood in which 2,3-DPG activity is reduced.[91] The clinical phenomenon has also been observed in septic patients and other critically ill patients.[92] An increased P_{50} means a decreased hemoglobin affinity for oxygen. This phenomenon has been observed in patients with chronic anemia.[93] The clinical application of P_{50} is not clear at present[94]; in fact, some doubt that there is any clinical usefulness for the measurement.[95]

Cyanosis

The term *cyanosis* indicates bluish coloration of the skin, mucous membranes, and nail beds, usually associated with an above-normal amount of reduced hemoglobin. Many studies have correlated cyanosis with the presence of 5 gm reduced hemoglobin per 100 ml blood. Other studies have revealed that the clinical detection of cyanosis varies widely with different observers and varying light conditions.[96] To the clinician, the presence of cyanosis must suggest a high probability of tissue hypoxia; however, the absence of cyanosis does not mean that there is no tissue hypoxia present. *Severe states of tissue hypoxia are possible without cyanosis.*

An increased number of red blood cells is called *polycythemia.* Polycythemia is most commonly associated with increased hemoglobin concentrations in the blood. Polycythemic states are also correlated to a high degree with chronic hypoxemic conditions.[13] Thus, it is not uncommon for a polycythemic patient who is hypoxemic to be cyanotic because of the presence of more than 5 gm reduced hemoglobin. However, because of the increased quantity of oxygenated hemoglobin per 100 ml of blood, there is usually adequate tissue oxygenation.

The clinical importance of cyanosis may be summarized by stating that its presence demands a careful and thorough clinical evaluation for the possibility of tissue hypoxia, whereas its absence should not be taken as an indication that adequate tissue oxygenation is present.

Intrapulmonary Shunting

A common cause of hypoxemia is a disease that produces intrapulmonary shunting (see Chapter 7). The physiologic (or total) shunt is that portion of the cardiac output that does not exchange with alveolar air.[2] The physiologic shunt has been subdivided into three components: (1) anatomic shunt, (2) capillary shunt, and (3) shunt effect (perfusion in excess of ventilation or venous admixture).

Anatomic Shunt

In the normal person approximately 2–5% of the cardiac output is returned to the left heart without entering the pulmonary vasculature.[2] This blood flow is via the bronchial, pleural, and thebesian* veins.[97] In addition to this normal anatomic shunt, pathologic anatomic shunts can exist, e.g., vascular lung tumors and right-to-left intracardiac shunts.

Capillary Shunt

Blood entering a pulmonary capillary that is coupled with an unventilated alveolus returns to the left heart without gaining oxygen. In other words, *capillary shunting is a result of pulmonary capillary blood in contact with totally unventilated alveoli.*

The sum of the anatomic and capillary shunts is frequently called the true or *absolute shunt*. This absolute shunt may be "refractory" to manipulation of oxygen therapy (see Chapter 15).

Shunt Effect

This physiologic defect is often referred to as *venous admixture* or *perfusion in excess of ventilation*. It occurs in an alveolar-capillary unit that has either a poorly ventilated alveolus or an excessive rate of blood flow.[98] Blood leaving this unit has a lower oxygen content than blood leaving a normal alveolar-capillary unit.[99]

This shunting secondary to ventilation/perfusion inequity is an extremely complex and variable component of the physiologic shunt. Its clinical importance is that it is responsive to oxygen therapy; that is, small increases in inspired oxygen concentration frequently result in dramatic increases in the amount of oxygen carried by the blood (see Chapter 15).[10]

A change in the characteristic of the alveolar-capillary membrane may act as an impedance to oxygen transfer from the alveolus to the pulmonary capillary. This defect in oxygen diffusion responds to oxygen therapy in a manner similar to ventilation/perfusion inequities.[135] Therefore, it is extremely difficult in the clinical setting of acutely ill patients to differentiate primary diffusion defects from inequities in ventilation/perfusion ratios. However, it should be remembered that the pathophysiology of each is distinctly different and should not be confused.

---

*The minor or lesser venous drainage of the myocardium. The major veins empty into the coronary sinus and thus the right atrium. The minor system empties directly into the ventricles.

The calculation of the physiologic shunt is described in detail in Chapter 19.

Physiologic Causes of Hypoxemia

Venous blood that does not exchange effectively with alveolar air always enters the arterial system with a lower oxygen content than the blood that has effectively exchanged. In the case where an absolute shunt exists, the blood enters the arterial system essentially unchanged from pulmonary artery blood. This desaturated hemoglobin mixes with the "effective" oxygenated blood, and arterial hypoxemia results in the equilibrium process.

This intrapulmonary shunting is the most common physiologic manifestation of pulmonary disease and is usually responsible for the arterial hypoxemia accompanying pulmonary disease. However, *it is incorrect to assume that all hypoxemia is caused by increased intrapulmonary shunting alone;* limited cardiovascular capability (i.e., limited ability to increase cardiac output) is often associated with significant hypoxemia.* Therefore, in patients with excellent cardiovascular reserve, it is possible to have a significant increase in shunting and minimal arterial hypoxemia. The physiologic causes of hypoxemia may be simplified and categorized into the following three major areas (Table 9–2).

Decreased Alveolar Oxygen Tensions

This results in decreased pulmonary capillary oxygen tensions secondary to reduced oxygen gradients, automatically leading to decreased arterial oxygen tensions. These regional areas of inadequate ventilation (because of uneven distribution of ventilation) are among

TABLE 9–2. – THE PHYSIOLOGIC CAUSES OF HYPOXEMIA

1. Decreased PA_{O_2}
   a. Hypoventilation
   b. Breathing less than 21% oxygen
   c. Underventilated alveoli (venous admixture)
2. Increased absolute shunt
3. Decreased mixed venous oxygen content
   a. Increased metabolic rate
   b. Decreased cardiac output
   c. Decreased arterial oxygen content

*This concept is explained further in the development of the shunt equation (see Chapter 19).

the most common causes of hypoxemia. This phenomenon has been referred to as *shunt effect, venous admixture,* or *ventilation/perfusion inequality.*

Increased Absolute Shunt

This pathophysiologic cause of hypoxemia is the result of totally unchanged venous (pulmonary artery) blood mixing with saturated blood. This type of arterial hypoxemia is often severe and "notably refractory" to oxygen therapy (refractory hypoxemia).

Decreased Mixed Venous Oxygen Content

Any mechanism that causes more oxygen extraction in the systemic capillaries may result in more desaturated hemoglobin in the venous blood. Therefore, the simultaneous presence of any degree of intrapulmonary shunting will result in an eventual decrease in arterial oxygen content if no compensatory mechanisms interfere. In other words, *the effect of any intrapulmonary shunt upon the arterial oxygen tension is directly related to the degree of desaturation of the venous blood that is being shunted.* There are three major causes for mixed venous blood having decreased oxygen content:

Increased metabolic rate (see Chapter 6).—Higher oxygen consumption leads to a lowered mixed venous oxygen content unless the organism is able to effectively compensate by increasing the cardiac output.

Decreased cardiac output.—This phenomenon is the most common cause of decrease in mixed venous oxygen content. Less blood flow per unit time through the capillary bed requires a greater degree of oxygen extraction per unit volume of blood if the tissue oxygen consumption is to remain unchanged.

Decreased arterial oxygen content.—This is most often secondary to an existent hypoxemia or to a significant anemia. Once again, the organism's primary compensatory mechanism is dependent upon increased cardiac output.

Cardiopulmonary Compensation for Hypoxemia

The Chemoreceptors

The peripheral chemoreceptors are small clusters of nervelike tissue located in the arch of the aorta and the bifurcation of the internal and external carotid arteries. They are referred to as the *carotid and aortic bodies.*[100] This small tissue mass has an exceptionally high metabolic rate and a very large blood supply—it is these properties that make them exceptionally sensitive to any decrease in oxygen supply[3]. Thus, when the chemoreceptors' oxygen tension drops for any reason (such as decreased arterial oxygen content, decreased arterial oxygen tension, or decreased blood flow) the response is to initiate afferent (sensory) signals to the brain. Efferent (motor) signals are then sent to the pulmonary system, which responds by increasing the total ventilation. The goal is that the increased ventilation resulting in an increased alveolar oxygen tension will in turn lead to a greater blood oxygen tension and content, thereby relieving the chemoreceptor stimulus. The peripheral chemoreceptors also play an important role in stimulating the heart in response to decreased oxygen supply.[3]

The Pulmonary Response to Hypoxemia

Normally the 159 mm Hg oxygen tension in inspired air results in an ideal alveolar gas oxygen tension of 101 mm Hg (this assumes an alveolar CO_2 of 40). In general, the alveolar oxygen tension rises as the degree of effective alveolar ventilation increases. The efficiency of this compensatory mechanism is limited in two major ways:

1. The mechanism has minimal effect on hypoxemia secondary to absolute shunting inasmuch as the blood that is effectively exchanging with alveolar air is already adequately oxygenated. In other words, the slight increase in alveolar oxygen tensions adds little content to the capillary blood that is exchanging and obviously has no effect on the shunted blood.

2. A point is reached, especially with large increases in total ventilation, at which the increased oxygen consumption due to the increased work of breathing negates any gain in available oxygen for general tissue utilization.

As a general rule, increasing inspired oxygen concentrations (up to 50–60%) by oxygen therapy is a far more efficient method of increasing alveolar oxygen tension (see Chapter 15). While this method does not require any increased ventilatory work, its effectiveness is still limited by the presence of any absolute shunt.

The Cardiac Response to Hypoxemia

The single most important compensatory mechanism available to the body to correct hypoxemia is increasing cardiac output. This concept may be more easily understood if it is assumed that the body's metabolic demand for oxygen is held constant. (Remember, it is not necessary in clinical practice for this assumption to exist.) If the cardiac output increases while the metabolic rate is stable, the amount of oxygen extracted from any given quantity of blood decreases. The effect of this mechanism is to increase the venous oxygen tension and the amount of hemoglobin still saturated with oxygen.

When hypoxemia is due to intrapulmonary shunting, the effect of the shunt on arterial blood is dependent upon the degree of desaturation of the shunted blood. As shown in Table 9–3, the heart may com-

TABLE 9–3.—CARDIOPULMONARY COMPENSATION FOR HYPOXEMIA

Table of values at 10 gm% hemoglobin and pH 7.40

P_{O_2} (mm Hg)	250	150	100	60	45	37	31	27	23
S_{O_2}%	100	100	98	90	80	70	60	50	40
Content (vol%)	14.1	13.8	13.4	12.4	11.0	9.7	8.3	7.0	5.6

1. Normal shunt, ventilation, cardiac output, metabolic rate

$$\dot{Q}s/\dot{Q}T = 5\% \quad P_{A_{O_2}} \text{ 100 mm Hg} \quad S\bar{v}_{O_2} \text{ 70\%}$$
$$95\% \ \dot{Q}c \text{ at } 13.4 \text{ vol\%}$$
$$5\% \ \dot{Q}s \text{ at } \underline{9.7 \text{ vol\%}}$$

$$C_{a_{O_2}} = 13.2 \text{ vol\%}$$
$$S_{a_{O_2}} = 97\%$$
$$P_{a_{O_2}} \text{ 95 mm Hg}$$

2. Increased shunt, normal ventilation, cardiac output, metabolic rate

$$\dot{Q}s/\dot{Q}T = 10\% \quad P_{A_{O_2}} \text{ 100 mm Hg} \quad S\bar{v}_{O_2} \text{ 70\%}$$
$$90\% \ \dot{Q}c \text{ at } 13.4 \text{ vol\%}$$
$$10\% \ \dot{Q}s \text{ at } \underline{9.7 \text{ vol\%}}$$

$$C_{a_{O_2}} = 13.0 \text{ vol\%}$$
$$S_{a_{O_2}} = 95\%$$
$$P_{a_{O_2}} \text{ 72 mm Hg}$$

3. Decreased cardiac output, normal shunt, ventilation, metabolic rate

$$\dot{Q}s/\dot{Q}T = 5\% \quad P_{A_{O_2}} \text{ 100 mm Hg} \quad S\bar{v}_{O_2} \text{ 50\%}$$
$$95\% \ \dot{Q}c \text{ at } 13.4 \text{ vol\%}$$
$$5\% \ \dot{Q}s \text{ at } \underline{7.0 \text{ vol\%}}$$

$$C_{a_{O_2}} = 13.0 \text{ vol\%}$$
$$S_{a_{O_2}} = 95\%$$
$$P_{a_{O_2}} \text{ 72 mm Hg}$$

4. Increased shunt, cardiac output; normal ventilation and metabolic rate

$$\dot{Q}s/\dot{Q}T = 10\% \quad P_{A_{O_2}} \text{ 100 mm Hg} \quad S\bar{v}_{O_2} \text{ 80\%}$$
$$90\% \ \dot{Q}c \text{ at } 13.4 \text{ vol\%}$$
$$10\% \ \dot{Q}s \text{ at } \underline{11.0 \text{ vol\%}}$$

$$C_{a_{O_2}} = 13.2 \text{ vol\%}$$
$$S_{a_{O_2}} = 97\%$$
$$P_{a_{O_2}} \text{ 95 mm Hg}$$

5. Increased shunt, oxygen therapy; normal cardiac output and metabolic rate

$$\dot{Q}s/\dot{Q}T = 10\% \quad P_{A_{O_2}} \text{ 250 mm Hg} \quad S\bar{v}_{O_2} \text{ 70\%}$$
$$90\% \ \dot{Q}c \text{ at } 14.1 \text{ vol\%}$$
$$10\% \ \dot{Q}s \text{ at } \underline{9.7 \text{ vol\%}}$$

$$C_{a_{O_2}} = 13.7 \text{ vol\%}$$
$$S_{a_{O_2}} = 100\%$$
$$P_{a_{O_2}} \ 140 \text{ mm Hg}$$

pensate for a shunt by increasing cardiac output. The venous hemoglobin saturation level is increased, and thereby the hypoxemic effect
of the shunted blood is decreased. Table 9–3 must be completely
understood in order to comprehend the clinical importance of cardiac
and pulmonary compensatory machanisms for hypoxemia. The following conditions are shown in the table:

    1.   Normal cardiopulmonary homeostasis.

    2.   Hypoxemia due to increased physiologic shunt.

    3.   Hypoxemia due to decreased cardiac output.

    4.   Increased physiologic shunt that is compensated by increased
cardiac output. Note that increased cardiac output results in increased
mixed venous oxyhemoglobin saturation.

    5.   Increased physiologic shunt compensated by oxygen therapy.

    In conclusion, it is necessary to understand the clinical manifesta-
tions of cardiac and pulmonary compensatory mechanisms for hypoxemia. It must be stressed once again that intrapulmonary shunting and
its effect on arterial hypoxemia cannot always be equated as a sole
cause and effect.

10 / Metabolic Acid-Base Balance

FEW SUBJECTS in clinical medicine have such an aura of confusion and mystification as does acid-base balance. As discussed in Chapter 2, to reflect the acid-base balance one must measure at least two of the three Henderson-Hasselbalch parameters, i.e., pH, plasma bicarbonate concentration (HCO_3^-), and plasma carbonic acid concentration (H_2CO_3). The pH can be directly measured (see Chapter 4) and the carbonic acid concentration can be indirectly obtained by measuring the dissolved carbon dioxide (PCO_2) in the plasma (see Chapter 2). Thus, by measuring these two (pH and PCO_2), the third (plasma bicarbonate concentration) can be calculated. Figure 3–3 reviews carbon dioxide transport and illustrates the fact that the ratio of plasma bicarbonate concentration (primarily controlled by the kidneys) to plasma carbonic acid concentration (primarily controlled by the lungs) determines the pH.

Not many years ago the clinician could not readily measure any of these parameters. When serum electrolytes became available from the clinical laboratory, the clinician attempted to reflect acid-base status by electrolyte changes. Had he been given the choice, the clinician would have directly measured acid-base status; however, this was not possible, so he applied the available electrolyte measurements and attempted to *reflect* the acid-base status. This gave rise to a complex and bewildering "cult," which made acid-base balance appear to be confusing and difficult. Today, blood gas analysis is clinically available, and direct measurement of the acid-base status is a reasonably simple procedure.

Some fifty years ago, pH and PCO_2 measurements became reasonably available to the research physiologist. At that time clinical medicine had not advanced to the point of cardiopulmonary supportive care and, therefore, the importance of effective ventilation and cardiopulmonary homeostasis was not appreciated. The overwhelming interest was in acid-base balance; thus the nomenclature for *all* abnormalities (metabolic or respiratory) was developed in terms of acid-base balance. For this reason, blood gas measurements have been *traditionally* interpreted in relation to the acid-base state. In this chapter, the significant metabolic (nonrespiratory) factors that regulate acid-base balance are discussed.

The Clinical Significance of Acid-Base Balance

Intracellular metabolism requires a very narrow range of free hydrogen ion concentration (pH) within which enzymatic and biochemical processes may function efficiently and appropriately. In addition, such critical functions as myocardial electrophysiology, central nervous system electrophysiology, and cellular responses to endogenous and exogenous chemical compounds (e.g., hormones and drugs) require specific pH milieu. Significant deviations from these narrow ranges (especially when they occur over short intervals of time) are poorly tolerated and may be life threatening. Therefore, an understanding of the homeostatic mechanisms working to maintain the normal pH is essential.

Regulation of Blood Acids

A *volatile* substance is one that is capable of chemically varying between the liquid and gaseous states. The major blood acid is carbonic acid (H_2CO_3).[101] Being a volatile acid it is controlled by the ventilatory system and will be discussed in detail in the following chapter.

All other potential sources of hydrogen ions can be considered nonvolatile (or fixed) acids and therefore under the major control of the kidneys, albeit the liver is also a major organ of metabolism. Figure 10–1 shows the major sources of nonvolatile acids: (1) dietary acids, (2) lactic acids, and (3) keto acids.

Dietary Acids

The normal food intake processed in the gastrointestinal tract tends to result in the absorption and metabolism of protein, which produces inorganic acids.[13] This tendency toward an "acidic" diet means that organic acids will also accumulate. The kidneys must be relied upon for excreting the 50–100 mEq of organic and inorganic acids generated per day. A normal diet in the presence of inadequate kidney function will result eventually in *renal acidosis*.

Lactic Acid

A normal production of lactic acid occurs in red and white blood cells, skeletal muscle, and brain.[13] Under normal circumstances this lactic acid is circulated in the blood and metabolized primarily by the liver and excreted by the kidneys.

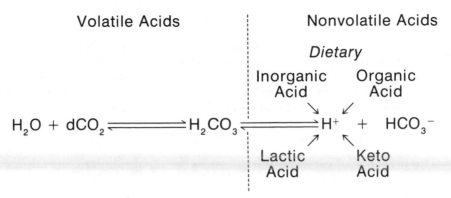

Fig 10–1. — Major sources of blood acids.

When adequate tissue oxygen is unavailable (hypoxia), metabolism must continue utilizing biochemical pathways that do not require oxygen. Such *anaerobic* (non-oxygen-utilizing) pathways produce a lactate ion and a hydrogen ion as end products. When these ions enter the blood they form lactic acid — a nonvolatile acid.

Lactic acidosis is the metabolic acidosis resulting from an accumulation of lactate ion and its accompanying hydrogen ion. The physiologic solution to this accumulation of lactic acid is the reestablishment of aerobic metabolism, which results in the lactate being metabolized primarily in the liver, with carbon dioxide and water as the ultimate metabolites.

Keto Acid

Normal aerobic metabolism utilizes the carbohydrate *glucose* ($C_6H_{12}O_6 + 6O_2 \rightarrow 6CO_2 + 6H_2O$). *Insulin* is necessary for the utilization of glucose by the cell. When glucose is not available, alternate aerobic pathways are used in which *keto acids* are the end products.

When cellular glucose is unavailable because of a lack of insulin, the resulting ketoacidosis is called *diabetic acidosis*. Ketoacidosis can result from starvation as well as from insulin deficiency.

Ketoacidosis is resolved by providing adequate amounts of glucose to the cell. In starvation this would mean glucose administration; in the diabetic it would mean insulin and glucose administration. When normal metabolic pathways are resumed, the keto acids are recycled through the normal pathways in which carbon dioxide and water are the metabolites.

Regulation of Blood Base

The primary blood base is plasma bicarbonate. Figure 3–3 indicates how bicarbonate ion is added or subtracted with a change in blood CO_2 content. However, this change is small and insignificant in comparison with the effect of the renal mechanism. Hydrogen ion is produced in the renal tubular cells by the following reaction:

$$CO_2 + H_2O \overset{CA}{\rightleftharpoons} H_2CO_3 \rightleftharpoons HCO_3^- + H^+.$$

The presence of carbonic anhydrase in the renal tubular cells allows the reaction to take place rapidly and completely (see Chapter 2).

Renal Mechanism

It is the *total* amount of hydrogen ion secreted that is significant to acid-base balance, and therefore the urine buffers play an important role in the kidney's ability to secrete large amounts of hydrogen ion.

The single most important urine buffer is *phosphate*. In glomerular filtrate 80% of the phosphate is in the dibasic form ($HPO_4^=$). In the urine 99% of the phosphate is monobasic ($H_2PO_4^-$); this means that great amounts of hydrogen ion can attach to phosphate and not change the urine pH. Ammonium is another important buffer. *The time required for the kidneys to significantly affect blood pH is a matter of hours.* This is in contrast to the respiratory mechanism, which can make significant changes in seconds.

The renal mechanism is shown schematically in Figure 10–2. The steps are as follows:

Step 1. — Urine starts as glomerular filtrate and has the same ionic concentrations as plasma. Therefore the bicarbonate ion concentration equals the plasma concentrations. Hydrogen ion will attach to bicarbonate ion *first*. This means that bicarbonate ion is essentially moved from urine to blood and, in the process, a hydrogen ion is excreted.

Step 2. — When no more bicarbonate ion is present in the urine, hydrogen ion attaches to dibasic phosphates. Again, for each hydrogen ion secreted, a bicarbonate ion is added to the blood.

Step 3. — Under certain circumstances ammonium ions may be excreted.

Essentially, for each hydrogen ion secreted into the urine the blood gains a bicarbonate ion. *It is this ability to add bicarbonate to the blood that is the kidney's main role in acid-base balance.*

BASIC PHYSIOLOGY OF BLOOD GASES

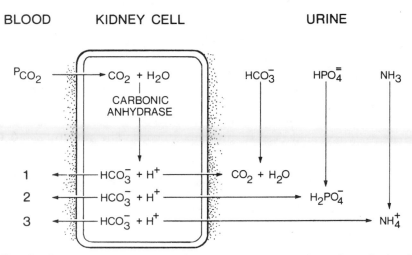

Fig 10–2.—Renal mechanism for blood base manipulation. Carbonic anhydrase exists in the kidney tubular cells and catalyzes the production of bicarbonate (HCO_3^-) and hydrogen ion (H^+) in quantities that are partly dependent on the blood P_{CO_2}. *(1)* Hydrogen ion combines with urine bicarbonate to produce carbon dioxide and water. The carbon dioxide is absorbed into the blood; the water is excreted in the urine. *(2)* Hydrogen ion attaches to dibasic phosphates and is excreted in the urine as $H_2PO_4^-$. *(3)* Under some circumstances the kidney excretes ammonium ion (NH_4^+). In all these cases a bicarbonate ion is added to the blood for each hydrogen ion secreted.

Electrolyte Mechanisms

The distribution of potassium ion (K^+) within intracellular and extracellular spaces influences acid-base balance.[101] Most of the potassium is intracellular, and if it leaves the cell it must be replaced by a hydrogen ion from the extracellular fluid (plasma).[8] Thus, *potassium leaving the cell will, in effect, add a bicarbonate ion to the plasma.*

In addition, potassium can be exchanged in the distal tubules of the kidney. This may have a significant effect on acid-base balance in certain circumstances.

Chloride ion (Cl^-) is freely exchangeable in the kidney tubules; this is not true for most other anions (e.g., phosphates) which are "fixed" and will not freely exchange.[13] When chloride ions are not available in sufficient quantity, cation exchange at the renal tubular level may be affected because of the lack of freely exchangeable anion.

Further, the total electrolytes must be in electrical balance. The primary electrolytes are:

CATIONS	ANIONS
Na^+	Cl^-
+	+
K^+	HCO_3^-

Thus, if the cations are normal, a reduction in chloride ion necessitates an increase in bicarbonate ion.[8]

The necessity for electric neutrality may produce electrolyte changes when acid-base disturbances occur. The meaning and the importance of the electrolyte changes are much easier to interpret when the acid-base status is known.

Renal Response to Acid-Base Imbalance

Metabolic alkalemia.—Increased plasma bicarbonate levels mean that some bicarbonate may actually be excreted in the urine. Thus, *the kidney may excrete base in response to excess blood base.*

Metabolic acidemia.—Decreased plasma bicarbonate means decreased urine bicarbonate ion. Thus, more bicarbonate is added to the blood as H^+ is excreted with phosphates. In other words, there is less of step 1 and more of step 2 in Figure 10–2.

Respiratory acidemia.—Increased P_{CO_2} causes increased hydrogen ion excretion by the renal tubular cells. This adds base to the blood.

Respiratory alkalemia.—Decreased P_{CO_2} causes decreased hydrogen ion excretion. Thus, less base is added to the blood.

Standard Bicarbonate

The clinical laboratory routinely includes some measurement of bicarbonate ion when reporting serum electrolytes. This is usually a measurement of *standard bicarbonate*—the plasma bicarbonate concentration after the blood has been equilibrated to a P_{CO_2} of 40 mm Hg.[102] The standard bicarbonate has traditionally been considered a reflection of the nonrespiratory, or metabolic, acid-base change. However, the standard bicarbonate does not quantify the degree of abnormality of the buffer base, nor does it consider the actual buffering capacity of the blood. In addition, it becomes confusing because *actual* plasma bicarbonate levels are now calculated directly from pH and P_{CO_2}.

Base Excess/Deficit

A far more satisfactory and clinically useful way to reflect the non-respiratory portion of acid-base balance is the calculation of base excess.[136] This calculation is an attempt to quantify the patient's *total base excess or deficit*, so that clinical treatment of metabolic acid-base disturbances can be aided. The calculation is made from the measurement of pH, Pa_{CO_2}, and hematocrit (inasmuch as the red blood cells contain the major blood buffers).[6] It is reported as milliequivalents per liter (mEq/L) of base above or below the normal buffer base range. Thus, a metabolic acidosis would have a *minus* base excess and is reported as such; e.g., a base excess of -10 mEq/L. A minus base excess is often referred to as a *base deficit*. The addition of nonvolatile acids affects the base excess, while changes in carbonic acid concentration do not change the buffer base. Thus, base excess is a true *nonrespiratory* reflection of acid-base status.[102]

In treating metabolic acid-base disturbances, it may be desirable to partly correct the metabolic abnormality in a short period of time. In the case of metabolic acidosis, this is most commonly accomplished by the intravenous infusion of sodium bicarbonate ($NaHCO_3$). Metabolic alkalosis is most commonly treated by: (1) correcting the underlying electrolyte imbalance (e.g., potassium or chloride); (2) using ammonium chloride (NH_4Cl) in a manner similar to that described for sodium bicarbonate; and (3) infusing dilute solutions of hydrochloric acid.

Calculation of Base Deficit

It is helpful to have a readily available means of estimating a safe amount of sodium bicarbonate that can be rapidly given to partly correct a metabolic acidosis. The measurement of base deficit allows the clinician to do just that, in accordance with the following steps:

1. A reasonable estimate of extracellular water can be made by dividing the normal body weight, in kilograms, by 3. This gives an estimate of the patient's extracellular water, in liters.

2. The base excess is reported in milliequivalents per liter, and the extracellular water in liters is now known. Thus, the total base excess can be calculated by multiplying the result of step 1 by the base excess.

3. Because this is only an estimate and the pathophysiology involved may be infinitely complex, one-half the calculated dose is rap-

TABLE 10–1.–THE HENDERSON-HASSELBALCH
PARAMETERS AND THEIR LABORATORY
NORMAL RANGES

	pH	$pH \propto \dfrac{[HCO_3^-]p}{Pco_2}$ Pco_2 (mm Hg)	$[HCO_3^-]p$ (mEq/L)
Normal	7.35–7.45	35–45	22–28
Acidotic	<7.35	>45	<22
Alkalotic	>7.45	<35	>28

idly administered intravenously. Blood gas measurements should be repeated in 15–20 minutes and the acid-base status again evaluated.

Example: A 90-kg man in metabolic acidosis has a base excess of −10 mEq/L. We calculate:

$$30 \text{ L} \times 10 \text{ mEq/L} = 300 \text{ mEq base deficit}$$

Therefore, 150 mEq sodium bicarbonate may be rapidly administered intravenously and blood gases repeated in 15 minutes. Severe acidemia may require vastly larger quantities of sodium bicarbonate than these calculations would suggest.[103]

It must be remembered that bicarbonate (and base excess) results are *not* measurements. Rather, they are *calculations* and are only as reliable as the accuracy of the pH and Pco_2 measurements upon which they are based.

Metabolic Acid-Base Interpretation

Blood gas studies provide us with all three Henderson-Hasselbalch parameters (Table 10–1). If normal ranges are known and the Henderson-Hasselbalch equation is understood, metabolic acid-base interpretation becomes a straightforward exercise.

Blood pH measurement determines *acidemia* and *alkalemia*—an excess or deficit of free hydrogen ion activity in the arterial blood. The pathophysiologic states of *acidosis* and *alkalosis* are determined by the calculation of blood acid and blood base.

The following is a list of the standard nomenclature in regard to metabolic acid-base imbalance. The arrows indicate depressed or elevated values; N means normal; and BE is base excess.

NOMENCLATURE	pH	PCO_2	$[HCO_3^-]p$	B.E.
METABOLIC ACIDOSIS				
Uncompensated (acute)	↓	N	↓	↓
Partly compensated (subacute)	↓	↓	↓	↓
Completely compensated (chronic)	N	↓	↓	↓
METABOLIC ALKALOSIS				
Uncompensated (acute)	↑	N	↑	↑
Partly compensated (subacute)	↑	↑	↑	↑
Completely compensated (chronic)	N	↑	↑	↑

11 / Respiratory Acid-Base Balance

IN NORMAL MAN it is estimated that metabolism produces approximately 12,000 mEq of hydrogen ion per day; less than 1% of this acid is excreted via the kidney.[13] This should be readily understood since the normal metabolite is carbon dioxide, a substance transported as a volatile acid (H_2CO_3) and excreted via the lung. Clinicians noted many years ago that acid-base imbalance is not life threatening for several hours to days following renal shutdown but becomes critical within minutes following the cessation of breathing. This essential role of *respiration* in the moment-to-moment maintenance of acid-base balance was fully appreciated more than sixty years ago.[104] Since increases in blood carbon dioxide content (increased PCO_2) cause increases in blood hydrogen ion concentration, the phenomenon was called *respiratory acidosis;* conversely, decreases in blood carbon dioxide cause decreases in blood hydrogen ion concentration, thus the term *respiratory alkalosis.* Table 11 – 1 denotes the criteria for the traditional nomenclature of *respiratory acidosis* and *respiratory alkalosis.*[105, 106]

There would be little purpose in changing this traditional nomenclature if it continued to adequately serve the modern clinician. In our opinion this has not been the case for the past two decades, primarily due to advances in the technologic ability to monitor cardiopulmonary function (ECG monitor, arterial blood gases, central venous pressure, Swan-Ganz catheterization, etc.) along with the improved capability

TABLE 11 – 1. – TRADITIONAL RESPIRATORY
ACID-BASE NOMENCLATURE*

NOMENCLATURE	pH	PCO_2	$[HCO_3^-]p$	BE
RESPIRATORY ACIDOSIS				
Uncompensated (acute)	↓	↑	N	N
Partly compensated (subacute)	↓	↑	↑	↑
Compensated (chronic)	N	↑	↑	↑
RESPIRATORY ALKALOSIS				
Uncompensated (acute)	↑	↓	N	N
Partly compensated (subacute)	↑	↓	↓	↓
Compensated (chronic)	N	↓	↓	↓

*Arrows indicate depressed or elevated levels; N is normal; and BE is base excess.

of supporting and correcting cardiopulmonary malfunction (fluid and electrolyte therapy, cardiovascular pharmacology, ventilator care, oxygen therapy, etc.).

Respiratory acid-base imbalance is primarily a ventilatory malfunction! Modern critical-care medicine demands that the malfunction in respiration be specifically diagnosed, monitored, and supported, especially the differentiation of ventilation from oxygenation. Thus, we contend that a modern view of respiratory acid-base balance must be developed based upon cardiopulmonary physiology and clinical application.

Organ System Failure

A generally acceptable definition of organ failure is "the failure of an organ system to meet the metabolic demands of the body."[9] In keeping with this definition, *heart failure* may be considered the failure of the heart to meet the metabolic demands of the body. This concept makes no reference to the cardiac output; that is, nothing is mentioned about whether the heart is putting out more blood, less blood, or the usual amount of blood. And in fact high-output cardiac failure is not only possible but quite common.

In terms of cardiopulmonary homeostasis, heart failure refers only to the relationship between metabolic demand and the ability of the heart to meet that demand. The measurement of cardiac output does not provide an objective measurement of physiologic adequacy, and therefore the clinical diagnosis of heart failure must be a matter of clinical judgment and deduction. This is true only because a single clinical objective measurement is not available.

The failure of the kidneys to meet the body's metabolic demands is called *renal failure*. As with heart failure and cardiac output, the measurement of urine output is not always diagnostic: high-output renal failure does exist. Fortunately, certain laboratory measurements (blood urea nitrogen, creatinine) may be used to diagnose and follow the course of renal failure. For this reason the clinical judgment of renal failure is far less subjective than is the assessment of heart failure.

Respiratory Failure

Respiration has been defined for almost 100 years as the movement of gas molecules across permeable membranes.[107] Although respiration may surely fail to meet metabolic demands at the internal as well as the external level (see Chapter 5), clinical tradition and practicality dictate that the term *respiratory failure* denote failure of adequate gas exchange at the pulmonary level.[1] Accepting this statement, we may define respiratory failure as *failure of the pulmonary system to meet the metabolic demands of the body.* This logically leads to the clinical assumption that *respiratory failure* means the lungs are inadequately providing oxygen and/or carbon dioxide exchange.

As such, respiratory failure is a broad and poorly delineated *clinical diagnosis* that makes no pretense of specifying or quantifying the pathophysiology. The limitations of such a clinical diagnosis are that it does not *document, specify,* or *quantitate* the disease process. The clinician attempts to accomplish these things through laboratory testing and other means. The following are several examples to illustrate this vitally important concept.

Acute Myocardial Infarction and the Electrocardiogram

A 40-year-old man enters the emergency room complaining of severe chest pain radiating to the left arm, shortness of breath, tachycardia, and "thready" pulse. He is clinically diagnosed as having an acute myocardial infarction. Of course, other diagnoses may be entertained, but acute myocardial infarction is certainly a reasonable clinical diagnosis. One important laboratory test would be the 12-lead electrocardiogram because: (1) it may *document* the clinical diagnosis of acute myocardial infarction; (2) it may further *specify* the insult (e.g., localize the area of injury); and (3) it may *quantitate* the insult so that serial measurements may be used to follow the course of the disease.

The term *acute myocardial infarction* is a useful and legitimate clinical diagnosis; however, *acute inferior wall injury* is an electrocardiographic diagnosis that documents, specifies, and quantitates the clinical diagnosis.

Acute Respiratory Failure and Blood Gas Measurement

1. A 60-year-old man enters the emergency room complaining of shortness of breath. He is tachypneic, tachycardic, sweaty, and cyanotic. A diagnosis of acute respiratory failure is made and several laboratory tests are ordered (arterial blood gases, chest x-ray, and so on). Arterial blood gas results show the PCO_2 is well below normal, the pH is alkalemic, and the arterial PO_2 is very low.

The blood gases have *documented* the gas exchange inadequacy (respiratory failure), *specified* this inadequacy to be a primary oxygenation problem, and *quantified* the severity of the gas exchange abnormality. The clinical diagnosis of acute respiratory failure is appropriate but limited. The arterial blood gases have documented, specified, and quantitated the physiologic insult and will lead to appropriate supportive measures if properly interpreted and applied.

2.   A 60-year-old man enters the emergency room with complaints similar to the man in the example above. Again, a diagnosis of acute respiratory failure is appropriately made. Arterial blood gases reveal a very high P_{CO_2}, a low pH, and a moderately low P_{O_2}.

The blood gases have *documented* acute respiratory failure, *specified* the pathophysiology as primarily ventilatory, and *quantitated* the severity of the insult. Surely this information will lead to different supportive care than in the previous example of respiratory failure.

The concept of respiratory failure is limited in its clinical usefulness and application — it must be accepted only as a general and nonspecific diagnosis. Arterial blood gas measurements are mandatory to document, specify, and quantitate the physiologic insult. Most importantly, one must differentiate primary oxygenation deficiencies from primary ventilatory deficiencies.

Oxygenation versus Ventilation

Tissue oxygenation may be considered the prime factor in the cellular life process. Logically, tissue oxygenation has traditionally been considered the prime function of the pulmonary system.[5] For this reason *respiratory failure* has traditionally been thought of primarily in terms of tissue oxygenation.

Chapters 6 and 9 have demonstrated how complex and difficult the clinical assessment of tissue oxygenation can be, even when precise blood gas measurements are available. This means that the assessment of respiratory failure in terms of tissue oxygenation must be a completely subjective clinical judgment. In addition, subtle clinical signs are easily missed, making respiratory failure a clinically unreliable diagnosis short of obvious extremis. Experience teaches that clinical evaluation of respiratory failure is far more difficult, unreliable, and unpredictable than the clinical evaluation of heart failure. In addition, tissue oxygenation may be totally unrelated to lung function; hypoxia can exist in many circumstances where the pulmonary system is functioning adequately.

Ventilation and oxygenation must be considered two separate entities! However, a complicated interrelationship exists between them. A significant change in one may affect the other — the extent of the effect is variable and complex, depending on the capabilities of the reflex mechanisms and the work capacities of the cardiopulmonary system. It is very important to clinically distinguish between ventilation and oxygenation, because the proper application of supportive modalities (e.g., oxygen therapy and ventilator care) depends on this distinction.

The Concept of Ventilatory Failure

The adequacy of alveolar ventilation is directly reflected in the arterial P_{CO_2}. Even though the disease state causing abnormal alveolar ventilation may have its etiology outside of the pulmonary system, we are still dealing with the inability of the pulmonary system to meet the metabolic demands as far as carbon dioxide is concerned.

If the physiologic assessment of the pulmonary system is considered in terms of carbon dioxide homeostasis, the concept of *ventilatory failure* results.[108] Respiratory failure includes the assessment of oxygenation and ventilation. *Ventilatory failure involves ventilation only;* oxygenation is assessed separately.

Defining Ventilatory Failure

In Chapters 5 and 6 we have seen that the metabolic rate is reflected in the respiratory quotient (see Fig 5–1). The respiratory quotient (RQ) represents the relationship of gas exchange in the peripheral capillaries; for the amount of oxygen consumed, an amount of carbon dioxide is produced. The carbon dioxide is carried by the venous blood to the lungs, where the moment-to-moment control of arterial carbon dioxide tension is determined.

Alveolar ventilation (see Chapter 8) reflects how well the lungs meet the carbon dioxide metabolic demands of the body. If arterial carbon dioxide tensions are to remain normal, the air exchange in the alveoli being perfused must increase as carbon dioxide production increases. *The arterial carbon dioxide tension directly reflects the adequacy of alveolar ventilation; therefore it provides an objective measurement of physiologic lung function.* Blood gases give us the objective measurement with which to diagnose ventilatory failure.

Ventilatory failure is defined as the condition in which the lungs are unable to meet the metabolic demands of the body as far as carbon dioxide homeostasis is concerned. Because alveolar ventilation is a reflection of how well the ventilatory demand is being met, ventilatory failure is the condition of inadequate alveolar ventilation in relation to the metabolic rate. The diagnosis *cannot* be made without arterial blood gas measurement; it is made without regard to the arterial or tissue oxygenation state.

Respiratory Acidosis

Table 11–2 demonstrates that both *ventilatory failure* and *respiratory acidosis* are terms describing an increased arterial P_{CO_2}. In other words, *ventilatory failure and respiratory acidosis are the same thing!* In the modern care of the critically ill patient, the term *ventilatory failure* is preferred because it refers to the *primary* cardiopulmonary abnormality; that is, it refers directly to the physiologic function in need of support.

Acute Ventilatory Failure

If the arterial carbon dioxide tension rises, plasma carbonic acid must correspondingly increase in concentration (see Chapter 2). The increase in carbonic acid results in a drop in blood pH. The kidneys respond by excreting more hydrogen ion and thereby add more bicarbonate ion to the venous blood (Chapter 10). If given enough time, this renal mechanism will gradually correct the pH to near normal.

If the arterial carbon dioxide tension is suddenly increased from 40 mm Hg to 80 mm Hg, the pH changes from 7.40 to 7.20 – the pH change is an *immediate* reflection of arterial carbon dioxide change. This arterial carbon dioxide tension to pH relationship may be changed by renal mechanisms over a period of time.

Obviously, then, an arterial carbon dioxide tension change that is accompanied by an appropriate pH change must be a recent event; i.e., ventilatory failure (respiratory acidosis) accompanied by an acidemia must be an *acute* event.

Acute ventilatory failure (*acute* respiratory acidosis) is the presence of a high arterial carbon dioxide tension with acidemia. It is usually

TABLE 11–2.—NOMENCLATURE FOR
VENTILATORY ABNORMALITIES

RESPIRATORY ACIDOSIS =	VENTILATORY FAILURE
Acute (uncompensated)	Acute
Chronic (compensated)	Chronic
RESPIRATORY ALKALOSIS =	ALVEOLAR HYPERVENTILATION
Acute (uncompensated)	Acute
Chronic (compensated)	Chronic

accompanied by hypoxemia and must be considered a dire clinical emergency!

Chronic Ventilatory Failure

If ventilatory failure has existed for a period of time or has developed very gradually over a long period of time, it will not be accompanied by an acidemia. *Ventilatory failure is chronic when metabolic compensation of the acidemia has occurred.* In other words, *chronic* ventilatory failure (*chronic* respiratory acidosis) is a high arterial carbon dioxide tension with a near-normal blood pH.

The differentiation of acute and chronic ventilatory failure is of more than academic interest. Basic biochemical cellular processes are affected by *sudden* environmental changes far more than by gradual changes.[13] For example, cellular function is disrupted to a far greater degree by a sudden pH change than by the gradual development of that same pH change. Acute ventilatory failure is far more life threatening than chronic ventilatory failure, not only because an acidemia exists but also because the change has been sudden. *The severity of ventilatory failure must be judged by the degree of the accompanying acidemia.*

Alveolar Hyperventilation (Respiratory Alkalosis)

Disease states may affect the cardiopulmonary homeostatic schema in such a way that normal alveolar air exchange is insufficient to meet metabolic demands. The patient is stimulated to breathe more, and he will do so if he possesses the muscular power. This results in an *alveolar hyperventilation;* i.e., an arterial carbon dioxide tension below normal. Table 11–2 denotes that *alveolar hyperventilation* and *respiratory alkalosis* are both terms to describe a decrease in arterial carbon dioxide tension. The term *alveolar hyperventilation* is preferred in order to remain consistent with the concept of referring to the *primary* cardiopulmonary malfunction.

Acute and Chronic

The alkalemia accompanying a sudden decrease in arterial carbon dioxide tension reflects the acuteness of ventilatory change. Thus, *acute* alveolar hyperventilation (*acute* respiratory alkalosis) is the occurrence of a decreased P_{CO_2} with alkalemia, and *chronic* alveolar hyperventilation (*chronic* respiratory alkalosis) is the occurrence of a decreased P_{CO_2} with a near-normal pH.

Causes of Alveolar Hyperventilation

Numerous disease processes may result in alveolar hyperventilation (respiratory alkalosis). A meaningful approach is to consider that the decreased arterial carbon dioxide tension occurs in response to three general pathophysiologic states: (1) arterial oxygenation deficits severe enough to stimulate peripheral chemoreceptors (see Chapter 9); (2) metabolic acidosis severe enough to stimulate the peripheral and/or central chemoreceptors; and (3) abnormal stimulation of the ventilatory centers of the central nervous system.

Ventilatory failure (respiratory acidosis) is always a form of respiratory failure because carbon dioxide exchange is inadequate. However, alveolar hyperventilation (respiratory alkalosis) can be considered a form of respiratory failure only when it is the result of an oxygen exchange deficiency (arterial oxygenation deficit).

Causes of Ventilatory Failure

Almost any disease that is severe enough, or present in a patient with limited abilities to compensate, may result in ventilatory failure.[108, 109] Figure 11–1 outlines the essential factors that allow for adequate alveolar ventilation. Diseases affecting the efficiency of any of these factors may lead to ventilatory failure.

Breathing depends upon muscles expending energy to provide mechanical work.[110] A given amount of work will provide a given degree of physiologic ventilation under normal circumstances. If disease states affect the efficiency of the pulmonary system, additional work

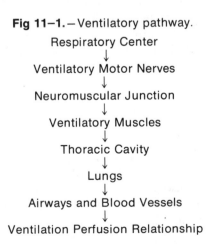

Fig 11–1.—Ventilatory pathway.

Respiratory Center
↓
Ventilatory Motor Nerves
↓
Neuromuscular Junction
↓
Ventilatory Muscles
↓
Thoracic Cavity
↓
Lungs
↓
Airways and Blood Vessels
↓
Ventilation Perfusion Relationship

may be necessary to accomplish adequate physiologic ventilation. Whether or not the organism can provide the additional work (and at what expense) is a question the clinician attempts to answer through the concepts of the work of breathing and ventilatory reserve.

Work of Breathing

Four major clinical factors must be considered when assessing the work of breathing: compliance, resistance, active expiration, and ventilatory pattern. It would be a disservice if the impression were left that quantification of the work of breathing is simple and straightforward.[111] The elastic recoil of the pulmonary system may be considered as if it were a single entity exerted primarily by the lungs with some assistance from the chest wall. Assuming this to be so, the concepts become simple. The *true* interrelationships and complexities of these mechanical factors are fortunately of little clinical significance, especially when dealing with patients in respiratory distress and possibly in need of mechanical support of ventilation. Therefore, it is clinically acceptable to view these factors in their simplistic relationships.

Compliance

In providing inspiration, the muscles of ventilation must expend enough energy to overcome: (1) the elastic recoil properties of the lung and chest wall and (2) airway resistance. It should be obvious that part of the energy expended for inspiration is "stored" in the elastic tissues as elastic recoil energy. This energy is normally used to provide most of the work of expiration.

In normal breathing at basal conditions, expiration is referred to as "passive" because it does not require active muscular work. The lower the compliance, the greater the elastic recoil energy available for expiration. The lower the compliance, the greater will be the energy expended to provide a deeper inspiration.

Resistance

To overcome increased airway resistance, during expiration an increased expenditure of energy may be needed. This increased expiratory energy is logically made available by deeper inspirations that allow for a greater degree of elastic recoil during expiration. This generally indicates that shallow breathing at a rapid rate demands a greater energy expenditure to overcome airway resistance than deep, slow breathing.

Active Expiration

Thus far, the discussion has assumed that expiration is entirely passive. As pointed out previously, this is the case in normal resting ventilation. In fact, in healthy people, expiration is almost totally passive, even with minute volumes as high as 20 L/min.[10] However, for very high minute volumes in patients with healthy lungs and for normal minute volumes in patients with diseased lungs, the expiratory muscles may be brought into play.[1, 5] That work must also be included in a total assessment of the work of breathing!

Ventilatory Pattern

If a constant minute volume is maintained, the work necessary to overcome elastic recoil is increased when breathing is deep and slow. On the other hand, the work expended to overcome airway resistance is increased when breathing is rapid and shallow. If total work is plotted against ventilatory frequency, *there is an optimal ventilatory frequency at which the total work of breathing is minimal* (Fig 11–2). Many investigators have noted that human subjects and animals tend to select ventilatory frequencies that correspond very closely to calculated frequencies for minimum work.[112] This response has also been well documented in patients with diseased pulmonary systems. When compliance is decreased, ventilatory frequency increases and tidal volumes decrease; when airway resistance increases, the ventilatory frequency decreases and tidal volumes increase. This is objective testimony to the clinical statement that *the ventilatory pattern present in a diseased patient is determined almost entirely by minimal expenditure of energy rather than by efficient physiologic ventilation!*[113] The ventilatory pattern chosen by a physiologically stressed patient must never be assumed to be advantageous in terms of molecular gas exchange; rather, it is the pattern requiring the least expenditure of energy for that minute ventilation.[5, 10]

Fig 11–2.–**a** is a graphic representation of the total work of breathing when minute ventilation is unchanged, but ventilatory pattern (tidal volume and frequency) is varied. Note that for any minute ventilation there is a ventilatory pattern that requires minimal work. Of course, total work is the summation of resistance work (airways) and elastic work (lung parenchymal and chest wall recoil forces).

If compliance is decreased, as in **b,** the graph shows that the pattern of ventilation at which the minute volume can be achieved with minimal work is dramatically altered.

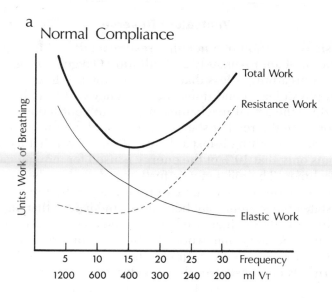

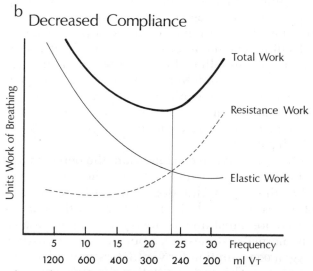

This is a schematic representation of the principle that work of breathing is the major factor determining ventilatory pattern (see text). (From Shapiro, B. A., Harrison, R. A., and Trout, C. A.: *Clinical Application of Respiratory Care* [Chicago: Year Book Medical Publishers, Inc., 1975].)

Ventilatory Reserve

A classic description of a healthy, resting adult includes an oxygen consumption of approximately 250 ml/min.[3] Oxygen consumption for the work of breathing is less than 5% of the total.[114] Even under these excellent physiologic conditions, the efficiency with which the energy is utilized for the actual mechanical aspects of ventilation is astoundingly poor.[115] In the resting state, about 90% of the energy expended for the work of breathing is lost as heat within the ventilatory muscles. This means only that 10% of the energy is used for moving gas in and out of the lungs. The efficiency is further reduced in the presence of pulmonary disease and with increased minute ventilation.[10] In severe disease states the system may become so inefficient that any oxygen potentially gained from increased ventilation is completely consumed by the increased muscular work.[111] This may progress to the point where an increase in ventilation results in net oxygen loss to the organism. In this circumstance, the alveolar gas improvement that can be accomplished by increased spontaneous ventilation is greatly limited.

The limitation of active ventilatory efficiency is reached only at very high minute volumes in healthy patients. However, in the presence of significant disease, the efficiency level may be so low as to impose severe limitations to even minor degrees of physiologic stress.[5] Despite the difficulties and numerous complexities that have been elaborated here, clinical guidelines for assessing ventilatory reserve have been developed.[2] The guidelines are based on functional concepts and clinical realities of the work of breathing. The following concept produces obtainable, reproducible, and reliable information that can be applied in the clinical circumstance of supporting gas exchange in the critically ill patient.

Of the body's total oxygen consumption, the percentage that is used by the ventilatory muscles is a reflection of the work of breathing.[111] If this is so, then the relationship depicted in Figure 11–3, A exists. As minute volume is increased, the percentage of the total oxygen consumption used for breathing is increased exponentially. In other words, in the normal resting state, a person uses approximately 5% of his total oxygen consumption for ventilatory muscular work.[116] As the person increases mechanical ventilation, he must use more muscular

---

Fig 11–3.—The work of breathing in relation to vital capacity (see text). In **B,** point *a* represents a VT of 500 ml with a Vc of 5 L; point *b* represents a VT of 500 ml with a Vc of 1 L.

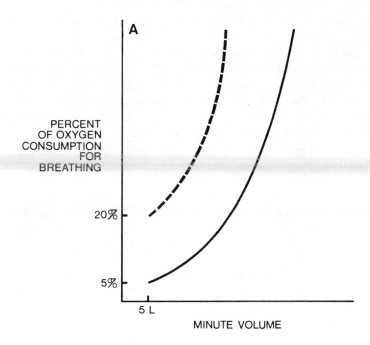

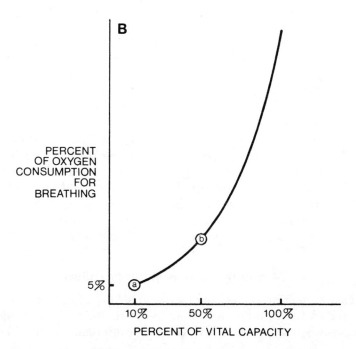

power. The increased muscular work demands increased oxygen consumption, and so the amount of total oxygen consumption used for the work of breathing increases. As a matter of fact, this increase in oxygen consumption is not linear; therefore, not only the amount but also the percentage of total oxygen consumption applied to the work of breathing increases. The untrained person has experienced this after running for a period of time; the work of breathing becomes so demanding that he must stop and, for a short period of time, concentrate on doing enough ventilatory muscular work to repay his oxygen debt.

Increasing minute ventilation causes an exponential increase in ventilatory oxygen consumption. If airway resistance is added, such as results from obstructive lung disease, the curve looks much like the dotted line in Figure 11-3, A. The work of breathing is far greater at the resting stage, and the increase in the percentage of oxygen consumption is far greater when there is increased airway resistance to overcome.

Figure 11-3, B shows the same curve plotted as a function of the vital capacity; that is, the curve represents the ventilatory work as a function of the portion of the vital capacity being used as tidal volume. Suppose, for example, that a man with a vital capacity of 5,000 ml has a tidal volume of 500 ml. He is using 10% of his vital capacity as tidal volume (a). The percentage of oxygen consumption being used for breathing is low. A second man has a vital capacity of only 1,000 ml but must maintain the same 500 ml tidal volume as the first man. He is using 50% of his vital capacity (b) and is consuming far more oxygen for breathing than the first man. It is important to note that even though the tidal volumes of both men are the same and the total body oxygen consumptions are the same, the percentage of oxygen consumed for the work of breathing is much higher for the second man.

In such an example, the second man has far less capability to increase his ventilation to meet stress. Because of his greatly diminished reserve, it is far more costly for him to increase his ventilatory work. *The greater the portion of the vital capacity that is being used for a high tidal volume, the less the ability of the patient to increase his tidal volume to meet a stressful situation. Therefore, vital capacity can be used as a gross indicator of ventilatory reserve.*

Pathogenesis of Ventilatory Failure

Diseases affecting the efficiency or capability of the various factors illustrated in Figure 11-1 may lead to ventilatory failure. In general, such diseases may be classified as cardiopulmonary, central nervous system, neurologic, musculoskeletal, hepatorenal, and fatigue. Ventilatory failure may be considered to follow a general pathophysiologic pattern regardless of its etiology.

Acute Ventilatory Failure

A sudden increase in the work of breathing or a sudden decrease in ventilatory reserves may result in the pulmonary system being incapable of meeting the normal carbon dioxide homeostatic demands. This may occur with little change in the clinical status; that is, factors such as pulse, blood pressure, breathing pattern, and alertness may change to minor degrees or *not at all!* Such a patient may imperceptibly go into acute ventilatory failure (acute respiratory acidosis) without significant clinical change until cardiopulmonary collapse ensues.

With acute ventilatory failure (acute respiratory acidosis) it is less important to understand the pathogenesis since the supportive and therapeutic care will be immediate and obvious. However, in chronic lung disease, a chronic ventilatory failure (chronic respiratory acidosis) often exists in which the understanding of its pathogenesis is crucial to its support and therapy.

Chronic Ventilatory Failure

There are three physiologic factors that lead to increased work of breathing in chronic obstructive pulmonary disease (COPD).

1.   An *increased functional residual capacity* means a constant state of hyperinflation which decreases the efficiency of air exchange at the alveolar level.[4] Thus, more ventilatory work is required to achieve adequate physiologic ventilation.

2.   Degenerative alveolar changes (emphysema) result in less area for exchange between alveolar air and pulmonary blood. Thus, a greater portion of the alveolar gas does not exchange with blood.[1] This "wasted" ventilation is called *deadspace ventilation*. Increased deadspace ventilation requires increased work of breathing.

3.   Bronchitic, asthmatic, and emphysematous diseases lead to *uneven distribution of ventilation,* creating hypoventilated areas in relation to blood flow.[12] This results in less than optimal oxygenation of the blood perfusing that area of lung. The shunt effect (venous admixture) leads to arterial hypoxemia, which causes the cardiopulmonary system to increase work in order to meet the organism's metabolic demands.

Increased work of breathing, decreased efficiency in the distribution of ventilation, decreased efficiency in the distribution of pulmonary perfusion, and hypoxemia lead to chronic carbon dioxide retention.

Figure 11–4 depicts the generalized pathogenesis of this ventilatory failure in chronic obstructive pulmonary disease. This teleologic discussion assumes the heart will not fail to meet the increased demands placed upon it. The early disease process results in a progressive arterial hypoxemia secondary to the ventilation-perfusion deterioration at point A. When the arterial oxygen tension reaches some minimal level B, usually around 60 mm Hg, the peripheral chemoreceptors experience decreased tissue oxygen supply and respond by stimulating both the ventilatory muscles and the myocardium.[3] This stimulation produces the amount of myocardial and ventilatory work necessary to maintain the arterial oxygen tension at a level minimizing chemoreceptor tissue hypoxia.

Maintaining the arterial oxygen tension at a level where the peripheral chemoreceptors are minimally stimulated in the face of progressive disease necessitates increasing ventilatory and myocardial work. The increasing ventilatory work is reflected in Figure 11–4 by a somewhat decreasing arterial carbon dioxide tension at C. The in-

Fig 11–4.—A theory on the pathogenesis of ventilatory failure in chronic obstructive pulmonary disease. A, decreasing arterial Po_2 due to early disease process; B, peripheral chemoreceptor stimulation begins and becomes the primary drive to breathe; C, arterial Po_2 level remains fairly constant while arterial Pco_2 level may decrease to some degree; D, theoretic points at which work of breathing is so costly that a decreased arterial Po_2 is unavoidable (see text); E, arterial Po_2 begins to decrease and arterial Pco_2 begins to increase.

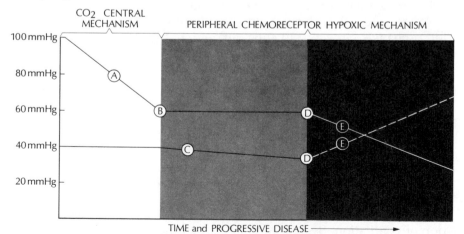

creased ventilatory and myocardial work continues to maintain the minimal arterial oxygen tension that "satisfies" the chemoreceptors.

Point D will be reached when the work of breathing uses so much oxygen that increasing total ventilation actually consumes more oxygen than is gained. In other words, physiologic deadspace is so great and shunting is so significant that a further increase in alveolar ventilation (seldom below 30 mm Hg) produces a net loss in arterial oxygen tension. It is essential to understand that at point D the organism faces a decrease in arterial oxygen tension, whether ventilation is unchanged, increased, or decreased, for the following reasons:

1. *Unchanged* alveolar ventilation leads to decreased arterial P_{O_2} because of increasing shunting and shunt effect.

2. *Increased* alveolar ventilation requires a great increase in ventilatory muscle work because the "wasted" ventilation (physiologic deadspace) is large. In addition, the vital capacity is decreased and airway resistance is increased. These factors lead to an oxygen consumption for increased ventilatory work that is greater than the oxygen gained from the increased alveolar ventilation.

3. *Decreased* alveolar ventilation decreases the oxygen consumed for the work of breathing, but this oxygen gain is not great enough to offset the oxygen loss from the decreased alveolar ventilation.

The organism obviously chooses the alternative that results in the smallest arterial oxygen loss for the least energy expended. As shown at points E in Figure 11–4, alveolar ventilation slowly decreases as arterial P_{O_2} slowly decreases. The cardiopulmonary homeostatic mechanisms dictate that the organism decreases effective ventilation and adjusts to the hypoxemia.[117] Recall that the organism chooses a ventilatory pattern according to work efficiency rather than ventilatory efficiency.

Summary

Respiratory failure is a useful clinical term referring to the failure of the pulmonary system to provide adequate gas exchange. Arterial blood gas measurements are necessary to document, specify, and quantitate the malfunction. The concept of ventilatory failure recognizes the physiologic malfunction as one of ventilation rather than the secondary effect of acid-base imbalance. By changing the focus from the general concepts of acid-base balance to a specific ventilatory function of the pulmonary system, a far more applicable and meaningful physiologic understanding is achieved in the clinical setting.

Clinical assessment of the ventilatory status is difficult and unreliable except *in extremis*. The difference between a patient with a given disease state manifesting alveolar hyperventilation or ventilatory failure may be the presence or absence of the muscular ability to increase total ventilation.

Pulmonary function studies alone are of minimal assistance because total ventilation does not necessarily reflect alveolar ventilation. For example, a high minute volume gives no information concerning alveolar ventilation unless the physiologic deadspace is known (see Chapter 8). A high minute volume and high physiologic deadspace may be thought of as "high-output ventilatory failure."

The diagnosis of ventilatory failure can be made only by arterial blood gas analysis! For example, a patient in status asthmaticus may have an unchanging disease state for several days. Due to lack of sleep and the great work of breathing, the patient may enter a serious fatigue state without showing any clinical signs of change. In other words, the patient may go imperceptibly from alveolar hyperventilation to ventilatory failure. This acute ventilatory failure (acute respiratory acidosis) increases in severity but becomes clinically obvious only in the extreme state when the patient is on the verge of cardiopulmonary collapse. The only way to reliably detect such subclinical, gradual, and critical ventilatory change is by serial blood gas measurement.

SECTION III

Interpretation of Blood Gas Measurements

MEDICAL PRACTICE is based on scientific knowledge whenever possible; however, much clinical knowledge is yet to be documented. Thus, for many centuries it has been recognized that medicine is an art as well as a science. The art of medicine is often referred to as *clinical judgment* or *clinical technique*. These terms mean that the clinician must attempt to base his actions on scientific factors as much as possible, but must understand that much of clinical practice is based on experience and clinical guidelines.

Clinical guidelines are generalizations that are not completely scientifically documented but have proved to be useful, dependable, and practical in the clinical setting. Such guidelines should be firmly based on scientific fact and modified by clinical application over a number of years. Clinical guidelines are not intended to be rigid or arbitrary; rather, they are meant to serve as sound guides for clinical practice. We believe the clinical guidelines in the following chapters are useful, dependable, and practical in applying arterial blood gas measurements to the critically ill patient.

12 / Guidelines for Interpretation

Laboratory Normal Ranges

MEASUREMENTS of a specific biologic function tend to be similar but not exactly identical in a given population. For example, a laboratory test performed on a large normal population will show a *range* of results—the variability within this range tending to be distributed in a symmetrical manner. Figure 12–1 graphically illustrates a symmetrical distribution; such a distribution is known as bell shaped. The *bell-shaped curve* represents the normal biologic system's usual distribution of variability in a particular measurement. In a perfect symmetrical distribution (a bell-shaped curve) the arithmetic average (the mean), the median (the middle number), and the mode (the number that appears most often) are all the same number. In a symmetrical distribution the *mean* represents the exact center of the population, with equal numbers above and below this center point.[118]

A computation can be made which includes approximately two thirds of the total population with the mean as the center. On a graph this includes two thirds of the area under the curve and is called *one standard deviation from the mean* (see Fig 12–1). *Two standard deviations from the mean* would include 95% of the total population, or 95% of the area under the curve with the mean as the center. In other words, two standard deviations from the mean would include all but 5% of the population—2½% on each extreme.

These statistical relationships are used in medical laboratories to establish "normal ranges." A *laboratory normal* is determined by performing these statistical calculations on a large series of measurements for a representative population. The computed mean is considered the laboratory normal value, with one or two standard deviations from the mean considered the normal ranges.[119] Remember, laboratory normal ranges are determined statistically after studying a large representative population.

pH and Pa_{CO_2} Laboratory Normals

The laboratory normal ranges for arterial carbon dioxide tension and pH are well documented and listed in Table 12–1.[120-122] These are universally accepted and must be memorized. Most clinical laboratories consider two standard deviations from the mean as the normal range since it includes 95% of the normal population.

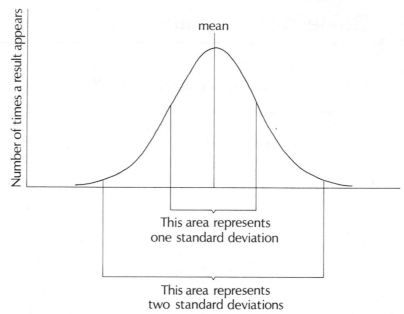

Fig 12–1.—A bell-shaped curve representing symmetrical distribution (see text). The mean represents the exact center of the population. One and two standard deviations from the mean are depicted.

Acceptable Therapeutic Ranges

For the clinician attempting to decide when to institute cardiopulmonary supportive measures or attempting to estimate cardiopulmonary homeostatic adequacy, it became obvious that small variations from the normal ranges of arterial carbon dioxide tension and pH are most often not clinically significant.[123, 124] This statement is no more than recognition of the fact that hospitalized patients requiring blood gas measurements are by and large seriously ill and are suspected of having various degrees of acid-base, ventilatory, or oxygenation abnormalities. Much discussion has taken place among physicians in respiratory care and critical-care medicine over such questions as:

TABLE 12–1.—LABORATORY
NORMAL RANGES

	MEAN	1 SD	2 SD
Pa_{CO_2} (mm Hg)	40	38–42	35–45
pH	7.40	7.38–7.42	7.35–7.45

TABLE 12-2.—ACCEPTABLE
THERAPEUTIC RANGES

Pa_{CO_2} (mm Hg)	30-50
pH	7.30-7.50

"At what pH abnormality should one intervene with supportive measures?"; or "How high must arterial carbon dioxide tension rise before mechanical support of ventilation should be seriously considered?". The past twenty years have taught these physicians that clinical therapeutic judgments are rarely influenced by minor variations from the normal ranges of arterial carbon dioxide tension and/or pH measurements.

It is from this clinical reality that the concept of "acceptable ranges" for arterial carbon dioxide tension and pH emerged (Table 12-2). These broader acceptable ranges are not attempts to replace the normal ranges; rather, they recognize that minor variations from normal in the seriously ill patient are seldom therapeutically significant. In the clinical application of blood gas measurement, these acceptable therapeutic ranges for arterial carbon dioxide tension and pH have proven dependable and practical. We shall use these ranges throughout the remainder of this text, hoping the reader will remember that we are not proposing that the normal ranges (see Table 12-1) be replaced or forgotten.

Our criteria for using the terms *acidemia, alkalemia, ventilatory failure,* and *alveolar hyperventilation* are listed in Table 12-3. These are clinical terms for blood gas interpretation and therefore are determined by clinically nonacceptable ranges of arterial carbon dioxide tension and pH.

Arterial Carbon Dioxide-pH Relationship

The pH is essentially the result of the plasma bicarbonate-plasma carbonic acid relationship (see Chapter 2). When acute changes in ventilation occur, a predictable relationship between pH and plasma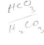

TABLE 12-3.—NOMENCLATURE FOR Pa_{CO_2} AND
pH OUTSIDE OF ACCEPTABLE RANGE

pH > 7.50	Alkalemia
pH < 7.30	Acidemia
Pa_{CO_2} > 50 mm Hg	Ventilatory failure (respiratory acidosis)
Pa_{CO_2} < 30 mm Hg	Alveolar hyperventilation (respiratory alkalosis)

TABLE 12-4.—APPROXIMATE
Pa_{CO_2}-pH RELATIONSHIP

Pa_{CO_2} (mm Hg)	pH	$[HCO_3^-]p$ (mEq/L)
80	7.20	28
60	7.30	26
40	7.40	24
30	7.50	22
20	7.60	20

carbonic acid results. This chemically represents the pH change due to variations in alveolar ventilation (Pa_{CO_2}), i.e., respiratory acid-base change. Although the relationship is not linear, within clinical ranges it is linear enough to assume an easy-to-remember guideline—when starting at an arterial P_{CO_2} of 40 mm Hg: for every 20 mm Hg increase in Pa_{CO_2}, the pH will decrease by 0.10 units; for every 10 mm Hg decrease in Pa_{CO_2}, the pH will increase by 0.10 units (Table 12-4). This guideline will prove helpful in quickly estimating the degree of abnormality that is due to *acute* ventilatory change.

Total Ventilation to Alveolar Ventilation Relationship

Chapter 8 discusses in detail the observation that total ventilation ($\dot{V}$) must be composed of a portion that respires—alveolar ventilation ($\dot{V}A$)—and a portion that does not respire—deadspace ventilation ($\dot{V}D$). Accepting minute ventilation (MV) as a measurement of total ventilation, the relationship may be written: $MV = \dot{V}A + \dot{V}D$.

It is well documented that in normal exercising man the physiologic deadspace either decreases or remains unchanged.[125] This results in the arterial carbon dioxide tension remaining the same or decreasing to a small degree. In other words, in normal exercising man alveolar ventilation does not change in relation to the metabolic rate because the metabolic rate and cardiac output have increased in a proportionate manner to the increase in ventilation.[126, 127]

The normal nonexercising man who is spontaneously hyperventilating is not well studied. One would expect the deadspace ventilation to increase as total ventilation increases because the cardiac output and metabolic rate would not be expected to increase in proportion to the total ventilation. An increase in deadspace ventilation is well documented in the hyperventilated patient on positive-pressure ventilation.[128, 129]

In patients with adequate cardiopulmonary reserves, clinical expe-

TABLE 12-5.—EXPECTED MINUTE VOLUME
TO ARTERIAL CARBON DIOXIDE TENSION
RELATIONSHIPS IN THE NORMAL
NONEXERCISING MAN

MV	Pa_{CO_2} (mm Hg)	RANGE (mm Hg)
Normal	40	35–45
Twice normal	30	25–35
Quadruple normal	20	15–25

rience has shown that diseases producing increases in minute ventilation without producing increases in physiologic deadspace result in a decreased arterial P_{CO_2}, e.g., pneumonia. The expected relationship between total ventilation and alveolar ventilation in these patients is shown in Table 12–5.

Many patients with adequate cardiopulmonary reserves manifest increases in total ventilation with an alveolar ventilation response less than that predicted in Table 12–5. It seems reasonable to assume that these patients may have increases in deadspace ventilation. Conversely, the patient who manifests a decreased alveolar ventilation (increased Pa_{CO_2}) without a decrease in total ventilation may be assumed to have an increased deadspace ventilation.

The guideline in Table 12–5 is a useful relationship for the spontaneously hyperventilating patient with adequate cardiopulmonary reserves. The existence of a significant *minute volume to PCO_2 disparity* should alert the clinician to the possibility that a deadspace-producing disease may be present (see Chapter 16).

Arterial Oxygen Tensions

In the healthy adult at sea level (760 mm Hg atmospheric pressure), the laboratory normal for arterial oxygen tension is usually stated as 97 mm Hg.[4, 120, 121] As with arterial carbon dioxide tensions and pH, minor variations in arterial P_{O_2} above 80 mm Hg seldom affect therapeutic clinical judgment. In addition, under most circumstances the oxygen saturation of hemoglobin is seldom significantly affected at a P_{O_2} above 80 mm Hg (see Chapter 9). Thus, we consider the acceptable therapeutic range for Pa_{O_2} at sea level as greater than 80 mm Hg (Table 12–6) and *hypoxemia is defined as an arterial PO_2 less than 80 mm Hg at sea level in an adult breathing room air.*

There are two major exceptions to this rule as shown in Table 12–6: (1) the normal newborn infant breathing room air usually has an arteri-

TABLE 12-6.—ACCEPTABLE ARTERIAL OXYGEN
TENSIONS AT SEA LEVEL BREATHING ROOM AIR
(21% OXYGEN)

ADULT AND CHILD	
Normal	97 mm Hg
Acceptable range	>80 mm Hg
Hypoxemia	<80 mm Hg
NEWBORN	
Acceptable range	40–70 mm Hg
AGED	
Acceptable range	
60 years old	>80 mm Hg
70 years old	>70 mm Hg
80 years old	>60 mm Hg
90 years old	>50 mm Hg

al oxygen tension range of 40–70 mm Hg;[130] and (2) the normal arterial oxygen tension levels decrease with age.[131] Lung degeneration is a normal part of the aging process and the alveolar degenerative processes are believed to cause hypoxemia.[132, 133] A general guideline is to subtract 1 mm Hg from the minimal 80 mm Hg level for every year over 60 years of age. This means that an arterial oxygen tension of 70 mm Hg in a 70-year-old patient and 60 mm Hg in an 80-year-old patient would be acceptable. The guideline is not applicable over 90 years of age.

Inspired Oxygen Concentration—Arterial Oxygen Tension Relationship ($F_{I_{O_2}}$–Pa_{O_2})

Hypoxemia is defined as an arterial P_{O_2} below an acceptable range *when breathing room air*. Oxygen therapy is a common feature in the treatment of patients who need blood gas analysis. A common question is: Should oxygen be withheld so that the patient can breathe room air during blood gas sampling? There is a widely held notion that a "room air blood gas" is essential as a baseline—this is not true! To withhold oxygen therapy from a hypoxemic patient until a blood gas sample is drawn is as wrong as withholding an anti-arrhythmic drug from a patient having serious ventricular arrhythmia until a complete 12-lead ECG is obtained. Although a room air baseline blood gas measurement is extremely helpful, it is by no means essential for the proper supportive care of the critically ill patient.

Increasing the inspired oxygen concentration by 10% means increasing the inspired oxygen tension by approximately 75 mm Hg (10% of 760 mm Hg). In the normal lung this means increasing the

TABLE 12-7.—THE GENERALIZED
INSPIRED OXYGEN-ARTERIAL
TENSION RELATIONSHIP*

FI_{O_2}	PREDICTED MINIMAL Pa_{O_2} (mm Hg)
30%	150
40%	200
50%	250
80%	400
100%	500

*If Pa_{O_2} is less than $FI_{O_2} \times 5$, the patient can be assumed to be hypoxemic at room air.

ideal alveolar oxygen tension by approximately 50 mm Hg.[4] Table 12-7 outlines an approximate relationship between inspired oxygen concentration and minimally acceptable arterial oxygen tensions in normal man. It is obvious that the minimally acceptable arterial P_{O_2} at each 10% rise in FI_{O_2} increases by approximately 50 mm Hg. A simple way to remember this is to multiply the FI_{O_2} by 5; the result will be a minimally acceptable P_{O_2} for that oxygen therapy. If that tension is not present, it may be assumed that the patient will be hypoxemic at room air.

13 / Clinical Approach to Interpretation

ALL BIOLOGIC SYSTEMS have limits beyond which they cannot function adequately. When cardiopulmonary homeostasis is stressed to its limit, the process of "dying" ensues; such uncompensated cardiopulmonary disease is reflected in blood gas measurements (see Chapter 5). These measurements can document, specify, and quantitate cardiopulmonary malfunction (see Chapter 11); however, the value of any laboratory measurements is dependent upon the ability of the physician, nurse, and respiratory care practitioner to apply them for the benefit of patient care. No matter how useful these measurements may be potentially, their actual benefit depends upon their clinical interpretation and application. One cannot expect to interpret the complex or unusual case without experience and special training. However, the situation need not be as confusing as it seems to most students, clinicians, and allied health personnel.

Based on the understanding of the material in the previous chapters, this chapter will outline and discuss a method of blood gas interpretation that is orderly, sensible, and reasonably simple. *The method is clinically very useful because the interpretation will delineate the primary life-threatening physiologic abnormality.* Furthermore, the interpretation will aid greatly in indicating the proper cardiopulmonary supportive measures needed. The interpretation also will allow subsequent blood gas measurements to guide the patient's continued supportive therapy.

Structured approaches to interpretation are necessary for the novice and useful to the initiated. Such categorized approaches are accepted in the teaching of radiologic and electrocardiographic interpretation, and they are no less applicable and necessary in the teaching of arterial blood gas interpretation.

Three basic steps should be followed when considering any set of blood gases:

Step 1: assessment of the ventilatory status. This will automatically lead to assessment of the metabolic acid-base balance when indicated.

Step 2: assessment of the hypoxemic state.

Step 3: assessment of the tissue oxygenation state.

Table 13–1 defines the clinical nomenclature used in this system.

133

TABLE 13-1.—NOMENCLATURE FOR CLINICAL
INTERPRETATION OF ARTERIAL BLOOD GAS MEASUREMENTS

CLINICAL TERMINOLOGY	CRITERIA
VENTILATORY FAILURE (respiratory acidosis)	Pa_{CO_2} above acceptable limit (50 mm Hg)
ALVEOLAR HYPERVENTILATION (respiratory alkalosis)	Pa_{CO_2} below acceptable limit (30 mm Hg)
Acute ventilatory failure	Pa_{CO_2} above acceptable limit (50 mm Hg), pH below acceptable limit (7.30)
Chronic ventilatory failure	Pa_{CO_2} above acceptable limit (50 mm Hg), pH within acceptable limits (7.30–7.50)
Acute alveolar hyperventilation	Pa_{CO_2} below acceptable limit (30 mm Hg), pH above acceptable limit (7.50)
Chronic alveolar hyperventilation	Pa_{CO_2} below acceptable limit (30 mm Hg), pH within acceptable limits (7.40–7.50)
ACIDEMIA	pH below acceptable limit (7.30)
ALKALEMIA	pH above acceptable limit (7.50)
ACIDOSIS	Pathophysiologic state where a significant base deficit is present (plasma bicarbonate below normal limit)
ALKALOSIS	Pathophysiologic state where a significant base excess is present (plasma bicarbonate above normal limit)

Step 1: Evaluation of the Ventilatory Status

The primary step in arterial blood gas interpretation should be to classify the carbon dioxide tension. This measurement is the direct reflection of the adequacy of alveolar ventilation. As shown in Table 13–2, the arterial carbon dioxide tension must be in one of three categories:

1. Less than 30 mm Hg: alveolar hyperventilation (respiratory alkalosis).

2. Between 30 and 50 mm Hg: acceptable alveolar ventilation.

3. Greater than 50 mm Hg: ventilatory failure (respiratory acidosis).

Assessment of the arterial pH in relation to the arterial carbon dioxide tension classification allows the determination of whether we are dealing with a primary ventilatory problem (respiratory acid-base imbalance) or a primary metabolic acid-base problem.

1. ALVEOLAR HYPERVENTILATION AND PH.—*a. Acute alveolar hyperventilation.*—With an arterial carbon dioxide tension below 30 mm Hg and the arterial pH above 7.50, adequate renal compensation has not been elicited and, therefore, the alveolar hyperventilation is assumed to be recent. The pH change is secondary to the ventilatory change.

TABLE 13-2.—EVALUATION OF VENTILATORY STATUS AND
METABOLIC ACID-BASE STATUS

CLASSIFICATION OF Pa_{CO_2}
Pa_{CO_2} < 30 mm Hg	Alveolar hyperventilation (respiratory alkalosis)
Pa_{CO_2} 30–50 mm Hg	Acceptable alveolar ventilation
Pa_{CO_2} > 50 mm Hg	Ventilatory failure (respiratory acidosis)

CLASSIFICATION OF VENTILATORY STATE IN CONJUNCTION WITH pH
1. Alveolar hyperventilation (Pa_{CO_2} < 30 mm Hg)
    a. pH > 7.50   *Acute* alveolar hyperventilation
    b. pH 7.40–7.50   *Chronic* alveolar hyperventilation
    c. pH 7.30–7.40   *Compensated* metabolic acidosis
    d. pH < 7.30   *Partly compensated* metabolic acidosis
2. Acceptable alveolar ventilation (Pa_{CO_2} 30–50 mm Hg)
    a. pH > 7.50   Metabolic alkalosis
    b. pH 7.30–7.50   Acceptable ventilatory and metabolic acid-base status
    c. pH < 7.30   Metabolic acidosis
3. Ventilatory failure (Pa_{CO_2} > 50 mm Hg)
    a. pH > 7.50   *Partly compensated* metabolic alkalosis
    b. pH 7.30–7.50   *Chronic* ventilatory failure
    c. pH < 7.30   *Acute* ventilatory failure

b. Chronic alveolar hyperventilation.—In the presence of alveolar hyperventilation, an arterial pH between 7.40 and 7.50 most probably represents a long-standing hyperventilation with renal compensation for the respiratory alkalemia; that is, the kidney has decreased plasma HCO_3^- to compensate for decreased H_2CO_3 (see Chapter 10). The primary physiologic problem is the ventilatory status change that is assumed to have existed for at least 24 hours.

c. Completely compensated metabolic acidosis.—Alveolar hyperventilation in the presence of an arterial pH between 7.30 and 7.40 probably reflects a primary metabolic acidosis in which the ventilatory system has normalized the pH by creating a respiratory alkalosis. It would be extremely unusual for this to represent a *primary* alveolar hyperventilation, inasmuch as this would mean the kidneys had overcompensated. *It is very unusual for either the renal system or the respiratory system to overcompensate.* It is a fairly safe clinical assumption that an alveolar hyperventilation accompanied by a pH of 7.30–7.40 is a completely compensated metabolic acidosis.

d. Partly compensated metabolic acidosis.—An alveolar hyperventilation in the presence of an arterial pH less than 7.30 usually does not represent a *primary* ventilatory change. This represents a primary metabolic acidemia to which the ventilatory system has responded by alveolar hyperventilating. Either the metabolic acidosis is very severe or the ventilatory system is incapable of doing the work necessary to completely compensate for the situation.*

2. ACCEPTABLE ALVEOLAR VENTILATION AND pH — *a. Metabolic alkalosis.* — An arterial carbon dioxide tension within an acceptable range accompanied by a pH greater than 7.50 most likely represents a primary metabolic alkalosis for which the ventilatory system has not compensated.†

b. Acceptable ventilatory and metabolic acid-base status. — An acceptable arterial carbon dioxide tension accompanied by an acceptable arterial pH must represent an acceptable ventilatory and acid-base state.

c. Metabolic acidosis. — An acceptable arterial carbon dioxide tension accompanied by an arterial pH less than 7.30 represents a metabolic acidosis for which the ventilatory system has not compensated.

3. VENTILATORY FAILURE AND pH. — *a. Partly compensated metabolic alkalosis.*‡ — An inadequate alveolar ventilation accompanied by an arterial pH greater than 7.50 probably represents a primary metabolic alkalosis for which the ventilatory system has partly compensated by producing an alveolar hypoventilation. In an alert patient whose central nervous system is intact, it is rare for the P_{CO_2} to rise above 60 mm Hg in response to metabolic alkalosis. However, in obtunded or comatose patients the P_{CO_2} may rise much higher.[134]

b. Chronic ventilatory failure. — An inadequate alveolar ventilation accompanied by a pH in the acceptable range probably represents a primary ventilatory change that has existed long enough for the renal mechanisms to have compensated.

c. Acute ventilatory failure — An inadequate alveolar ventilation accompanied by an arterial pH below 7.30 most probably represents an acute change in the ventilatory state.

Review of Step 1

At the completion of step 1 all blood gases must fall within one of

---

*Steps 2 and 3 may lead us to change this interpretation to alveolar hyperventilation if severe hypoxemia and hypoxia are present. This would be a lactic acidosis; i.e., a metabolic acidosis due to accumulation of nonvolatile blood acids.

†We shall see later that this interpretation may change when accompanied by hypoxemia. (See acute alveolar hyperventilation superimposed on chronic ventilatory failure, Chapter 15.)

‡This may represent acute alveolar hyperventilation superimposed on chronic ventilatory failure. Steps 2 and 3 will delineate this circumstance. (See Chapter 15.)

TABLE 13-3.—SEVEN PRIMARY BLOOD GAS CLASSIFICATIONS*

CLASSIFICATION	Pa_{CO_2}	pH	$[HCO_3^-]p$	BE
Primary ventilatory				
1. Acute ventilatory failure	↑	↓	N	N
2. Chronic ventilatory failure	↑	N	↑	↑
3. Acute alveolar hyperventilation	↓	↑	N	N
4. Chronic alveolar hyperventilation	↓	N	↓	↓
Primary acid-base				
1. Uncompensated acidosis	N	↓	↓	↓
Uncompensated alkalosis	N	↑	↑	↑
2. Partly compensated acidosis	↓	↓	↓	↓
Partly compensated alkalosis	↑	↑	↑	↑
3. Compensated alkalosis or acidosis	↑ or ↓	N	↑ or ↓	↑ or ↓

*Arrows indicate depressed or elevated values; N is normal; and BE is base excess.

the seven primary classifications outlined in Table 13–3. There are four primary ventilatory classifications and three primary acid-base classifications. In other words, after one step the basic differentiation has been made as to whether the clinical pathology is primarily cardiopulmonary or primarily acid-base and whether the process is acute or chronic.

It is essential that the methodology presented thus far be completely mastered. The following are sample blood gas results. The reader should test himself or herself as to the placing of these results in one of the seven primary classifications and should not proceed further in this chapter until this is completely mastered and understood.

Exercises

Do *not* attempt any correlation with clinical situations; simply interpret each set of values in accordance with step 1. For clarity, the units are omitted. They are understood to be:

Pco_2	mm Hg
Plasma bicarbonate (PBic)	mEq/L
Base excess (BE)	mEq/L

All values are arterial.

	1	2	3	4	5	6	7
pH	7.26	7.52	7.60	7.44	7.38	7.20	7.56
Pco_2	56	28	55	24	76	25	44
PBic	24	22	51	16	42	9	38
BE	−4	+1	+26	−6	+14	−17	+14

1. Acute ventilatory failure (acute respiratory acidosis).

2. Acute alveolar hyperventilation (acute respiratory alkalosis).
3. Partly compensated metabolic alkalosis.
4. Chronic alveolar hyperventilation (chronic respiratory alkalosis).
5. Chronic ventilatory failure (chronic respiratory acidosis).
6. Partly compensated metabolic acidosis.
7. Uncompensated metabolic alkalosis.

	8	9	10	11	12	13	14
pH	7.36	7.60	7.32	7.56	7.55	7.20	7.46
P_{CO_2}	25	25	95	40	58	78	26
PBic	15	24	49	34	49	30	18
BE	−10	+4	+15	+11	+20	0	−4

8. Completely compensated metabolic acidosis.
9. Acute alveolar hyperventilation.
10. Chronic ventilatory failure.
11. Uncompensated metabolic alkalosis.
12. Partly compensated metabolic alkalosis.
13. Acute ventilatory failure.
14. Chronic alveolar hyperventilation.

	15	16	17	18	19	20	21
pH	7.36	7.54	7.24	7.20	7.42	7.24	7.10
P_{CO_2}	83	29	60	38	28	28	95
PBic	48	24	26	15	18	12	29
BE	+15	+3	−2	−13	−5	−15	−5

15. Chronic ventilatory failure.
16. Acute alveolar hyperventilation.
17. Acute ventilatory failure.
18. Uncompensated metabolic acidosis.
19. Chronic alveolar hyperventilation.
20. Partly compensated metabolic acidosis.
21. Acute ventilatory failure.

	22	23	24	25	26	27	28
pH	7.39	7.48	7.40	7.24	7.54	7.55	7.24
P_{CO_2}	25	28	56	44	25	52	32
PBic	15	20	34	18	21	44	14
BE	−7	−1	+7	−7	0	+17	−13

22. Completely compensated metabolic acidosis.
23. Chronic alveolar hyperventilation.
24. Chronic ventilatory failure.
25. Uncompensated metabolic acidosis.

26. Acute alveolar hyperventilation.
27. Partly compensated metabolic alkalosis.
28. Uncompensated metabolic acidosis.

	29	30	31	32	33	34	35
pH	7.35	7.52	7.48	7.16	7.28	7.46	7.55
P_{CO_2}	25	48	20	83	20	58	20
PBic	14	39	16	29	9	40	18
BE	−11	+14	−7	−3	−17	+11	−3

29. Completely compensated metabolic acidosis.
30. Uncompensated metabolic alkalosis.
31. Chronic alveolar hyperventilation.
32. Acute ventilatory failure.
33. Partly compensated metabolic acidosis.
34. Chronic ventilatory failure.
35. Acute alveolar hyperventilation.

Step 2: Assessment of the Hypoxemic State

Evaluation of the hypoxemic state must *follow* evaluation of the ventilatory and acid-base status. Only by knowing the specific pathophysiologic state of the patient's ventilatory system and his acid-base status can one obtain any meaningful clinical information concerning arterial oxygen tensions.

The only direct information obtained from the arterial oxygen tension measurement is the indication of the existence or absence of *arterial hypoxemia*. Hypoxemia makes the existence of tissue hypoxia a distinct possibility, but does not assure its presence. Of equal importance is the fact that hypoxemia may be the *cause* of ventilatory and acid-base disturbances.

Arterial hypoxemia is an arterial oxygen tension less than the minimally acceptable limit (see Chapters 9 and 12). Table 12–6 lists the minimal normal values. These are values derived from normal subjects breathing room air, which means that the *actual diagnosis of hypoxemia can be made only when the patient is breathing room air,* however, hypoxemia may be assumed and evaluated while breathing enriched oxygen atmospheres. Table 13–4 lists the suggested ranges and nomenclature on room air and with oxygen therapy. Since many patients are already on oxygen therapy when blood gas samples are obtained, it is essential that the *probable hypoxemic state* be assessed so that the adequacy of the oxygen therapy can be evaluated. Even more important is to assess the effect the oxygen therapy is having on

TABLE 13-4.—EVALUATION OF HYPOXEMIA (STEP 2)

ROOM AIR; PATIENT UNDER 60 YEARS OLD

Mild hypoxemia	$Pa_{O_2} < 80$ mm Hg
Moderate hypoxemia	$Pa_{O_2} < 60$ mm Hg
Severe hypoxemia	$Pa_{O_2} < 40$ mm Hg

For each year over 60 years, subtract 1 mm Hg for limits of mild and moderate hypoxemia. At any age, a Pa_{O_2} less than 40 mm Hg indicates severe hypoxemia.

OXYGEN THERAPY

Uncorrected hypoxemia	$Pa_{O_2} <$ room air acceptable limit
Corrected hypoxemia	$Pa_{O_2} >$ room air minimal acceptable limit; < 100 mm Hg
Excessively corrected hypoxemia	$Pa_{O_2} > 100$ mm Hg; $<$ minimal predicted (Table 12-7)

the ventilatory status (see Chapter 15). Do *not* interrupt the oxygen therapy to assess hypoxemia; that is not necessary and may be dangerous.

1. **UNCORRECTED HYPOXEMIA.**—Despite increased inspired oxygen concentrations, the arterial P_{O_2} remains less than the room air minimal limits; i.e., it remains in the hypoxemic range. Any patient who is "room air hypoxemic" may have uncorrected hypoxemia with proper oxygen therapy. In other words, *uncorrected hypoxemia does NOT necessarily mean the oxygen therapy is inadequate.* Obviously, the tissue oxygenation state must be assessed before changing the oxygen therapy.

2. **CORRECTED HYPOXEMIA.**—This is the condition in which oxygen therapy has corrected the arterial hypoxemia; i.e., the oxygen therapy has restored the arterial P_{O_2} to an acceptable range. In this situation, hypoxemia must exist at room air, because the Pa_{O_2} is below the predicted normal level for that oxygen therapy.

3. **EXCESSIVELY CORRECTED HYPOXEMIA.**—This is the condition in which the Pa_{O_2} is greater than 100 mm Hg with oxygen therapy. Hypoxemia must exist at room air, because the Pa_{O_2} is not as high as one would expect with the administered FI_{O_2}. Too much oxygen is being administered: in most circumstances a Pa_{O_2} greater than 100 mm Hg is excessive. This usually indicates the need to reduce the oxygen delivered.

When the arterial P_{O_2} is greater than the theoretically minimal Pa_{O_2} for that FI_{O_2}, it means one of two things: (1) oxygen therapy may not be needed because hypoxemia may not exist, or (2) oxygen consumption is greatly reduced.

As stated in Chapter 9, arterial hypoxemia results from one of three physiologic causes: decreased alveolar oxygen tensions, increased absolute shunting, or decreased mixed venous oxygen content.

Exercises

The following exercises are specifically for learning and practicing step 2—assessment of the hypoxemic state. (Step 1 is necessarily a part of these exercises.) Do *not* attempt any correlation with clinical situations; simply interpret each set of values. For clarity the units are omitted. They are understood to be:

P_{CO_2}	mm Hg
Plasma bicarbonate (PBic)	mEq/L
Base excess (BE)	mEq/L
P_{O_2}	mm Hg
$F_{I_{O_2}}$	percent
Age	years

All values are arterial.

	1	2	3	4	5
pH	7.60	7.20	7.44	7.38	7.28
P_{CO_2}	25	78	24	76	20
PBic	24	30	16	42	9
BE	+4	0	−6	+14	−17
P_{O_2}	65	50	58	50	110
$F_{I_{O_2}}$	21	21	21	21	21
Age	30	45	40	70	35

1. Acute alveolar hyperventilation (acute respiratory alkalosis) with mild hypoxemia.
2. Acute ventilatory failure (acute respiratory acidosis) with moderate hypoxemia.
3. Chronic alveolar hyperventilation with moderate hypoxemia.
4. Chronic ventilatory failure with hypoxemia.
5. Partly compensated metabolic acidosis without hypoxemia.

	6	7	8	9	10
pH	7.48	7.54	7.48	7.24	7.46
P_{CO_2}	28	25	33	60	58
PBic	20	21	24	26	40
BE	−1	0	+1	−2	+11
P_{O_2}	65	90	85	50	59
$F_{I_{O_2}}$	21	21	50	21	21
Age	40	40	40	45	70

6. Chronic alveolar hyperventilation with mild hypoxemia.
7. Acute alveolar hyperventilation without hypoxemia.
8. Acceptable ventilatory status with corrected hypoxemia.
9. Acute ventilatory failure with hypoxemia.
10. Chronic ventilatory failure with hypoxemia.

	11	12	13	14	15
pH	7.24	7.42	7.54	7.16	7.36
P_{CO_2}	32	28	29	83	83
PBic	14	18	24	29	48
BE	−13	−5	+3	−3	+15
P_{O_2}	100	50	65	30	45
$F_{I_{O_2}}$	21	40	21	40	21
Age	40	50	45	40	80

11. Uncompensated metabolic acidosis without hypoxemia.
12. Chronic alveolar hyperventilation with uncorrected hypoxemia.
13. Acute alveolar hyperventilation with mild hypoxemia.
14. Acute ventilatory failure with severe uncorrected hypoxemia.
15. Chronic ventilatory failure with hypoxemia.

	16	17	18	19	20
pH	7.48	7.24	7.46	7.40	7.48
P_{CO_2}	33	28	26	56	33
PBic	24	12	18	34	24
BE	+1	−15	−4	+7	+1
P_{O_2}	75	90	70	55	50
$F_{I_{O_2}}$	50	21	21	21	50
Age	70	40	75	60	30

16. Acceptable ventilatory status with corrected hypoxemia.
17. Partly compensated metabolic acidosis without hypoxemia.
18. Chronic alveolar hyperventilation *without* hypoxemia
    (75-year-old person; minimal normal P_{O_2} is 65 mm Hg).
19. Chronic ventilatory failure with hypoxemia.
20. Acceptable ventilatory status with uncorrected hypoxemia.

	21	22	23	24	25
pH	7.48	7.55	7.26	7.56	7.10
P_{CO_2}	33	20	56	32	95
PBic	24	18	24	28	29
BE	+1	−3	−4	+6	−5
P_{O_2}	160	45	50	100	35
$F_{I_{O_2}}$	50	21	21	21	21
Age	30	40	40	40	50

21. Acceptable ventilatory status with excessively corrected hypoxemia.
22. Acute alveolar hyperventilation with moderate hypoxemia.
23. Acute ventilatory failure with hypoxemia.
24. Uncompensated metabolic alkalosis without hypoxemia.
25. Acute ventilatory failure with severe hypoxemia.

	26	27	28	29	30
pH	7.48	7.20	7.32	7.48	7.52
P_{CO_2}	20	25	95	20	28
PBic	16	9	49	16	22
BE	−7	−17	+15	−7	+1
P_{O_2}	90	100	40	90	55
F_{IO_2}	50	21	21	21	21
Age	30	40	75	50	40

26. Chronic alveolar hyperventilation with corrected hypoxemia.
27. Partly compensated metabolic acidosis without hypoxemia.
28. Chronic ventilatory failure with hypoxemia.
29. Chronic alveolar hyperventilation without hypoxemia.
30. Acute alveolar hyperventilation with moderate hypoxemia.

Step 3: Assessment of the Tissue Oxygenation State

The evaluation of the hypoxemic state is of critical importance in patient care and is essential to the application of proper supportive respiratory care. The need to evaluate the tissue oxygenation state (see Chapters 6 and 9) is likewise essential, and it cannot be separated from the hypoxemic evaluation. To accomplish the assessment of the tissue oxygenation state one must clinically assess (1) the cardiac status, (2) the peripheral perfusion status, and (3) the blood oxygen transport mechanism.

The assessment of cardiac output and microcirculatory perfusion is purely clinical; i.e., it depends upon vital signs and physical examination. Some key factors are blood pressure, pulse pressure, heart rate, ECG, skin color and condition, capillary fill, sensorium, electrolyte balance, and urine output. *If cardiac output and microcirculatory perfusion are adequate, only the blood oxygen transport mechanism can be interfering with proper tissue oxygenation.* This mechanism is composed of three factors: (1) arterial oxygen tension, (2) blood oxygen content, and (3) hemoglobin-oxygen affinity.

1. ARTERIAL OXYGEN TENSION.—The arterial oxygen tension (see Chapter 9) determines the initial oxygen blood-tissue gradient in the peripheral capillary. This gradient is an important factor in determining how fast, and for how long, oxygen will pass from blood to tissue.

Hypoxemia means the blood side of the pressure gradient is less than normal. This means that tissue hypoxia is quite probable. If hypoxia is to be avoided in the presence of hypoxemia, the cardiovascular system must provide an increased rate of tissue perfusion or an increased hemoglobin content (polycythemia) must be present (see Chapter 9).

2. **BLOOD OXYGEN CONTENT.** — The blood oxygen content (see Chapter 9) determines how much oxygen may leave the blood for a given decline in oxygen tension. This means it will be an important factor in determining how much oxygen may leave the blood before the pressure gradient is no longer adequate for blood-tissue exchange. As the arterial oxygen content decreases, there is a decrease in the amount of oxygen that may leave the capillary blood for any given decline in oxygen tension. If no increase in cardiac output occurs, the decreased oxygen content may result in insufficient oxygen delivery to the tissues. Factors affecting blood oxygen content are:

a. Hypoxemia, which results in decreased hemoglobin saturation (and thus a decreased oxygen content).

b. Hypercarbia, acidemia, and hyperthermia, which cause a hemoglobin curve shift to the right. This means the hemoglobin is less saturated at any given arterial oxygen tension.

c. Hypoxemia and acidemia, in combination, may drop oxygen contents to critically low levels. *Whenever hypoxemia and acidemia co-exist, tissue hypoxia should be assumed.*

d. Anemia obviously decreases oxygen content because there is less hemoglobin per 100 ml blood. Factors other than decreased hemoglobin content can cause this; among such factors are methemoglobinemia and carbon monoxide poisoning (see Chapter 3).

3. **HEMOGLOBIN-OXYGEN AFFINITY.** — Various factors affect the strength with which hemoglobin attaches to (and holds on to) oxygen molecules (see Chapters 3 and 9). This is important because *the greater the hemoglobin-oxygen affinity, the less effective is a given oxygen blood-tissue gradient in transferring oxygen to tissue.*

a. Alkalemia and hypothermia increase hemoglobin-oxygen affinity. This shift to the left may be very significant clinically when alkalemia co-exists with hypoxemia or a decreased oxygen content (see Chapter 9).

b. Lowered P_{50} means that at pH 7.40 the hemoglobin is 50% saturated at a Po_2 of less than 27 mm Hg; i.e., oxygen affinity is increased (see Chapter 9).

Evaluation of the tissue oxygenation state is not a simple task! It is a clinical evaluation process that is significantly enhanced with the proper interpretation of blood gas measurements.

14 / Guidelines for Sampling and Quality Control

ONE CANNOT APPROACH the subject of the clinical application of blood gas measurements without addressing the problems involved in obtaining the blood sample, preparing it for the laboratory, and assuring that the laboratory produces accurate and reliable results. Since statistically significant data from several medical centers are not available, we must depend upon guidelines that are reasonably documented and have evolved from five to ten years of clinical application. Most importantly, we must avoid anecdotes, case reports, and "rules of thumb" dictating our procedures and methods.

This chapter elucidates the guidelines and techniques used in the critical-care areas and central blood gas laboratory of Northwestern Memorial Hospital for over five years. This experience includes nearly half a million blood gas samples from the general hospital patient population; the medical, surgical, and neonatal intensive care areas; the operating rooms; and outpatients. We believe the criteria are well founded in the documented medical literature and consistent with the experience of numerous other medical centers. We present the material as *a right way* of obtaining, preparing, and measuring blood gas samples — by no means do we believe these are the *only* ways!

Obtaining the Sample

Blood has been used as a source of laboratory studies for many years because it reflects total body status and is readily available. Since the integrity of a vessel must be violated to obtain a blood sample, it is reasonable to be concerned about the problems that may develop from such an invasion. The three most significant problems are bleeding, obstruction of the vessel, and infection.

Venous puncture would have theoretically fewer problems than arterial puncture because: (1) the pressures are lower and therefore bleeding would be less of a problem, (2) venous collateral vessels are abundant so that obstruction of one peripheral vein is seldom a significant problem, and (3) interruption of venous flow is less significant to tissue viability than interruption of arterial flow. Thus, it is understandable how venous puncture and venous blood samples became the standard for laboratory blood tests.

Criteria for Site of Arterial Puncture

The reasons blood gas measurements must be made on arterial blood have been documented in great detail (Section II). Therefore, it is important to develop a rationale for deciding what criteria should be used to determine the appropriate sampling site and technique.

COLLATERAL BLOOD FLOW. — Arterial puncture may cause vessel spasm, intraluminal clotting, or bleeding with the formation of a periarterial clot (hematoma).[137-139] Any of these factors may result in diminution or total interruption of blood flow to the tissues normally supplied by that vessel. Therefore, an important consideration in choosing arterial puncture sites should be the potential collateral (alternative) blood flow available in the event the artery becomes obstructed.

Figure 14 – 1 illustrates the excellent collateral arterial blood supply that exists in the hands and feet. The *brachial artery* at the elbow has reasonable collateral flow when it becomes obstructed. However, there is no adequate collateral flow if the *femoral artery* becomes obstructed immediately below the inguinal ligament.

VESSEL ACCESSIBILITY. — It is easier to palpate, stabilize, and puncture a superficial artery than a relatively deep one. Superficial arteries are found at the distal ends of the extremities — areas that are commonly accessible in the outpatient as well as in the critically ill patient.

PERIARTERIAL TISSUES. — Muscle, tendon, and fat are reasonably insensitive to pain, whereas bone periosteum and nerves are very sensitive. Thus, arteries surrounded by relatively insensitive tissues are desirable so that the puncture can be as free from pain as possible. In addition, arteries that are not immediately adjacent to veins are preferable to minimize the chance of inadvertent venous puncture.

Radial Artery Puncture

The radial artery at the wrist meets the above criteria as being the safest and most accessible site for arterial puncture.[140] The vessel is located superficially at the wrist and is not adjacent to large veins. The collateral circulation is usually adequate via the ulnar artery. If puncture of the bony periosteum is avoided, the procedure is relatively pain-free.

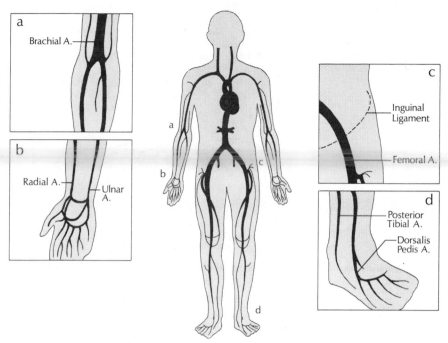

Fig 14–1.—Schematic of collateral circulation. **a,** deep brachial, superior, and inferior ulnar collateral arteries usually provide sufficient flow to the radial and ulnar arteries if the brachial artery is obstructed. **b,** the palmar arches usually provide adequate flow to the hand and fingers when either the ulnar or radial arteries are obstructed. **c,** the deep femoral artery is the only collateral source of flow to the lower extremity—it usually originates well below the level of the inguinal ligament; thus, obstruction to flow in the femoral artery above this point leaves the lower extremity without arterial blood flow. **d,** the arterial arches that provide blood flow to the foot and toes are usually supplied by both the dorsalis pedis and the posterior tibial arteries.

Puncture of the brachial artery in the antecubital fossa is a logical alternative when the radial arteries are unavailable. It is our opinion that routine arterial punctures by nonphysicians should be limited to the radial artery.

ALLEN'S TEST. — Although more complicated and refined methods of assessing collateral circulation exist,[141, 142] a simple, clinically reliable maneuver for assessing collateral circulation in the hand is Allen's test.[143] The hand is closed tightly to form a fist—this maneuver will force as much blood from the hand as possible. Pressure is then ap-

(a)

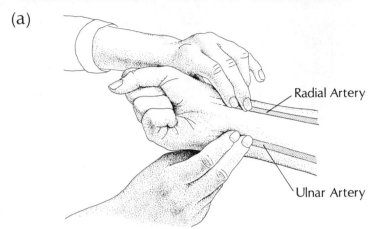

Radial Artery

Ulnar Artery

(b)

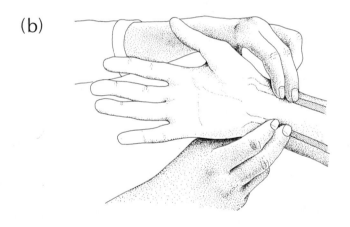

(c)

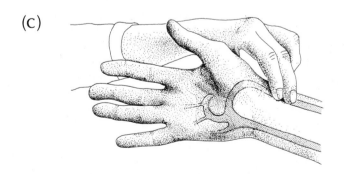

plied directly at the wrist, compressing and obstructing both the radial and ulnar arteries (Fig 14–2). The hand is then relaxed (but not fully extended), revealing a blanched palm and fingers.[144] The obstructing pressure is next removed from only the ulnar artery while the palm, fingers, and thumb are observed; they should become flushed within 15 seconds as the blood from the ulnar artery refills the empty capillary beds.[145] This flushing of the entire hand documents that the ulnar artery *alone* is capable of supplying the entire hand since the radial artery is still occluded. This result constitutes a positive Allen's test.

Under these circumstances it may be assumed that arterial puncture causing an obstruction of the radial artery will not result in diminution of blood supply to the hand. If the ulnar artery does not adequately supply the entire hand (a negative Allen's test), the radial artery should not be used as a routine puncture site for arterial blood gases.[146]

TECHNIQUE FOR RADIAL ARTERY PUNCTURE. — Most procedures can be accomplished safely and efficiently in many different ways. The following is a protocol we have found very successful in teaching radial artery puncture. We include this stepwise procedure as a prototype, realizing that numerous modifications may be made without affecting the skill or ease with which the procedure can be accomplished.

1.   The process is explained to the patient and the radial and ulnar arteries are palpated and followed by application of Allen's test.

2.   The skin at the puncture site is cleansed with an alcohol swab and the area examined for skin rash or other abnormalities that may rule out that site for needle puncture.

3.   A small skin wheal is raised with a local anesthetic through a 25-gauge needle. Experience has shown that the great majority of punctures are accomplished on the first attempt;[147] however, a skin wheal allows another attempt to be made without pain. In addition, most patients appreciate the fact that you are anesthetizing the area prior to needle insertion. There has been no evidence to substantiate the claim that slight breath holding or mild hyperventilation during the puncture significantly affects the blood gas results.

4.   The skin puncture and subsequent procedure should be done with the needle alone! This permits greater control and allows the

---

Fig 14–2. — Allen's test. **a,** the hand is clenched into a tight fist and pressure applied to the radial and ulnar arteries. **b,** the hand is opened (but not fully extended); the palm and fingers are blanched. **c,** removal of the pressure on the ulnar artery should result in flushing of the entire hand.

needle to be placed more parallel to the artery. We suggest a 20- or 21-gauge needle, however, any gauge (25–19) may be used without affecting the accuracy of the sample.[148]

5. The angle between the needle and the artery should be as small as possible. This makes the hole through the arterial wall oblique so that the circular smooth muscle fibers will seal the hole when the needle is withdrawn. Blood will appear at the hub of the needle when the artery is entered. If the needle goes completely through the artery, slowly withdraw the needle until its tip is once again within the lumen, as evidenced by free-flowing blood through the needle.

6. Attach the syringe. Don't be concerned about the small amount of blood lost; after using this technique several times, you will find there is very little loss of blood. Figure 14–3 shows the stability of the needle and syringe during the withdrawal of blood with this technique. If a plastic syringe is used you may have to pull slightly on the plunger to establish a free flow of blood.

The control gained by not having the syringe attached during the puncture allows observation of the blood flow, distinguishing pulsatile arterial flow from venous flow.

7. After 2–4 ml have been obtained, the needle is withdrawn and pressure is applied to the site for a minimum of two minutes. If the

Fig 14–3.—Radial artery puncture technique.

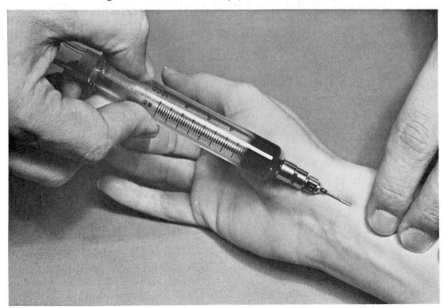

needle entry was oblique the incidence of hematoma (periarterial accumulation of blood) is rare.

Femoral Artery Puncture

The site that *least* fulfills the criteria for arterial puncture is the femoral artery below the inguinal ligament. This artery is deep under the skin and lies adjacent to a large vein and nerve. The limited collateral arterial flow makes obstruction a threat to the entire lower limb.

This site is popular primarily because the vessel is large. It is commonly believed that it is the easiest artery to puncture because of its size. With a little experience one can accomplish radial or brachial artery puncture more easily than femoral artery puncture.

Serious complications from arterial puncture usually involve femoral artery puncture.[149] *This should be the site of last resort!*

Arterial Cannulation

The past five years have seen a great deal of controversy over the placement of indwelling arterial cannulas for the immediate availability of arterial blood samples and continuous arterial pressure monitoring. Many physicians prefer that the nursing and therapy personnel do repeated single punctures to follow serial blood gas measurements. Often, the personnel responsible for drawing the blood gases are unable to maintain appropriate monitoring since it requires a great deal of time and effort. Most important, the samples are often difficult or impossible to obtain when they are needed most, i.e., during periods of cardiopulmonary instability. Of course, single punctures cannot provide continuous arterial pressure monitoring.

Our indication for placing an arterial line is when a patient is (or may become) cardiopulmonary unstable—in other words, any patient who needs serial blood gas monitoring and/or continuous arterial pressure monitoring. These general criteria for arterial lines are based upon their great contribution to the care of the critically ill patient—especially when compared to their low complication rate.

COMPLICATIONS.—Ultrasound flow studies of arteries that have been cannulated show a significant incidence of diminished or absent flow for limited periods of time.[150] Where adequate collateral circulation is present, these findings do not result in significant complication to the patient.[151,152] The most severe complications are necrosis and loss of tissue.[153] There have been several case reports of finger and toe loss, and numerous cases of lower limb loss or the necessity for femoral endarterectomy.[154-161]

Personal communication with more than a dozen critical-care centers throughout the country and recent publications reveal data similar to our experience[156-158] — of more than 5,000 consecutive arterial lines placed by our respiratory care service (none of them femoral), eight patients (less than 0.2%) have suffered necrosis of fingers or toes. These eight patients had either severe four-extremity perfusion deficit or primary vascular disease. None of these patients survived the critical illness.

Infection is a potential problem with all vessel cannulations.[162] Our incidence of systemic sepsis or local infection secondary to arterial cannulation is the same as for venous cannulation.[163,164] It can be stated that arterial lines properly cared for have no greater complication rate than that of indwelling venous catheters. We believe the placement of continuous arterial lines is well justified in the care of the critically ill patient.

TECHNIQUE FOR INDWELLING ARTERIAL CANNULA

I. *Equipment*
   A. Intravenous cannula, consisting of:
      2.5-ml syringe
      Teflon cannula
      Needle stylet
   B. 2.5-ml syringe, 25-gauge needle, 1 ampule 1% xylocaine
   C. Skin antiseptic swabs, sterile scalpel
   D. Continuous arterial keep-open setup, consisting of:
      1-ml ampule heparin (10 mg/ml)
      500-ml plastic transfer pack
      Intravenous tubing set
      Fenwal pressure bag
      2 fused sterile three-way stopcocks
      Intraflo flushing device (Sorenson)
      1-ft-high pressure tubing (Cobe)
II. *Continuous Arterial Keep-Open Technique*
      Note. — Have this prepared before insertion of the cannula.
   A. Add 10 mg (1 ml) heparin to 500 ml normal saline.
   B. *Important:* Absolutely no air bubbles can be present in the tubing or bag. Eliminate any bubbles by applying firm snapping pressure to the bag or tubing.
   C. Insert intravenous tubing into the transfer pack. Make sure that the drip chamber does not completely fill with solution.
   D. *Important:* Adhesive tape all junctions of the intravenous tubing so that no medication can be injected into the arterial line.
   E. Free the tubing of air; then shut off the tubing control and apply *150–300 mm Hg* of pressure from the Fenwal bag to the transfer pack. Maintain at least 50 mm Hg above systolic pressure.

F. Connect Intraflo to the intravenous tubing.

G. Attach three-way stopcocks, with 2.5-ml syringes attached, to the Intraflo. Be sure the stopcocks are "off."

H. Attach the Cobe tubing to the remaining end of the fused stopcocks and connect to the cannula.

I. Rid the entire setup of air and attach it to the arterial cannula (Fig 14–4).

III. *Puncture Technique with Intravenous Cannula*

    Note.— Follow the single-stick technique where indicated.

A. Prep the area with skin antiseptic.

Fig 14–4.—The continuous arterial keep-open technique. *a,* cannula entering radial artery; *b,* Cobe tubing; *c,* fused stopcocks; *d,* Intraflo device; *e,* intravenous tubing; *f,* Fenwal pressure bag; *g,* transfer pack with heparinized solution; *h,* aneroid pressure transducer (electronic transducer may be used).

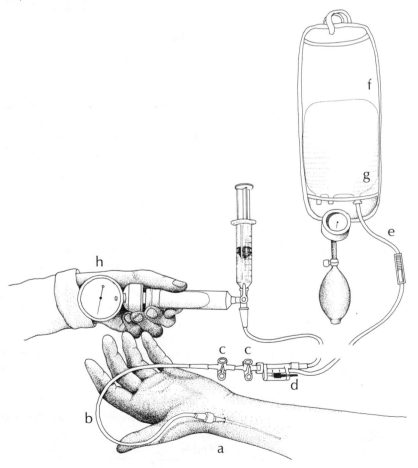

    B. Apply the local anesthetic, as in the single-stick technique.

    C. The skin overlying the vessel to be entered is cut with a scalpel.

    D. Follow the single-stick needle puncture technique, insert the Teflon cannula into the artery one-half its distance.

    E. When proper placement is obtained, secure the cannula to the skin and attach the arterial keep-open line.

    F. Apply antibacterial ointment to the puncture site.

    G. Suture, if necessary (which is seldom).

       The Intraflo device flushes approximately 3 ml/hr of the heparinized solution from the transfer pack.[165] This has proven to provide ample flushing to prevent the cannula from clotting. In addition, a tubing that connects to a pressure transducer can be attached directly to the Intraflo device.

IV. *Drawing a Blood Sample*

    A. A waste syringe is attached to the stopcock furthest from the cannula and solution is withdrawn until undiluted blood enters the syringe. Five to six times the tubing volume is advised.[166]

    B. Two milliliters of blood are drawn into the sample syringe through the other stopcock.

    C. The plunger is gently pulled on the Intraflo device until the blood is cleared from the tubing.

Capillary Samples

Clinical circumstances arise with infants and small children where arterial samples are either not readily available or not indicated. This situation occurs primarily in the well-perfused infant where Po_2 measurement is desirable but not to the point of warranting arterial sticks or cannulation.

In a well-perfused infant, arterialized capillary blood will show a consistent correlation with arterial Pco_2 and pH, and will reflect a *minimal* arterial Po_2 value. It must be emphasized that Po_2 data from capillary samples are meaningless in a baby whose perfusion status is not perfectly normal.[167-177] When cardiopulmonary instability exists, an arterial cannula is as indicated in the small child and infant as in the adult.[178-182]

TECHNIQUE FOR CAPILLARY SAMPLES.—1. A highly vascularized capillary bed (earlobe, heel, great toe, or finger) is chosen and warmed for 10 minutes by either heat lamp or warm towels.

2. A *deep* puncture is made with a scalpel blade so that a free flow of blood appears from the wound without squeezing the area. Squeezing will "de-arterialize" the sample.

3. A preheparinized capillary tube (75–100 μl) is inserted deep into the drop of blood. The blood should flow easily into the tube. Two capillary tubes provide an ideal sample.

4. The tubes should be immediately sealed and placed in ice.

TABLE 14–1.—VENOUS OXYGEN TENSION AND
OXYGEN CONTENTS FOR BLOOD RETURNING FROM
DIFFERENT ORGAN SYSTEMS*

ORGAN SYSTEM	Pv_{O_2} (mm Hg)	% SAT.	$[Ca_{O_2} - Cv_{O_2}]$(vol%)
Cerebral	37	69	6.3
Coronary	30	56	11.4
Intestinal	45	80	4.1
Renal	74	94	1.3
Skeletal muscle	32	60	8.0
Skin	75	95	1.0

*Conditions: Arterial Po_2 = 100, Ca_{O_2} = 20.2 vol%, Hb = 15 gm%,
cardiac output = 6 L/min, human subject at rest.

Venous Samples

Appropriately obtained samples of peripheral venous blood in well-perfused patients may be used to grossly reflect the arterial acid-base status.[183, 184] However, peripheral venous blood for assessing the oxygenation state is unacceptable. This is because the distribution of the total cardiac output to the various organ systems depends on the local arteriolar resistance and vasomotor tone within the respective capillary beds.[9] The cardiovascular system always attempts to maintain blood flow to critical organ systems at an optimal level. This is accomplished by appropriate adjustments in cardiac output and changes in regional resistances. Therefore, the various organ systems do not necessarily receive a blood supply proportional to their metabolic demands.

The net effect is differing degrees of oxygen extraction from the blood supplied to the respective organ systems. Therefore, the values of venous oxygen tension would vary depending on the organ system from which the venous sample was taken. These differences exist under basal resting conditions and become even more exaggerated in the critically ill patient. Table 14–1 lists the variations in venous blood gas measurements for blood returning from different organ systems under basal resting conditions.[5, 10]

Pulmonary Artery Samples

These samples are obtained from a pulmonary artery catheter and are discussed in chapter 20. When blood samples are aspirated from these catheters, the sample must be withdrawn *slowly*.[185] Rapid aspiration can result in pulmonary capillary blood being mixed with the pulmonary artery blood. This would cause dramatic increases in oxygen content.

Preparing the Sample

Errors in blood gas measurement may be due to improperly obtaining or handling the sample prior to delivery to the laboratory.

Glass versus Plastic Syringes

Early studies suggested that plastic substances absorb so much oxygen that the use of plastic syringes for blood gas samples would be ill advised. More recent studies have not substantiated these assumptions.[186] In essence, pH and P_{CO_2} values are not affected, whereas P_{O_2} values for samples in excess of 400 mm Hg drop more rapidly in plastic than in glass syringes.[187] It is doubtful that this circumstance is clinically significant.

We *prefer* glass syringes for the following reasons: (1) the barrel has minimal friction with the syringe wall and the pulsating arterial pressure is clearly visible as the blood fills the syringe; (2) there is seldom a need to "pull back" on the barrel, a maneuver that can cause air bubbles to enter the sample around the barrel; and (3) small air bubbles adhere tenaciously to the sides of a plastic syringe, making it difficult to expel the air from the samples.[188]

Although glass is preferred, there is no *strong*, valid objection to the use of appropriate plastic syringes. In fact, we routinely use plastic syringes for sample collection from arterial lines.

Anticoagulants

When blood is removed from a vessel the clotting mechanisms immediately are activated. This results in a sample of serum plus a blood clot. Blood gas measurements must be accomplished on "whole blood," i.e., unclotted and unseparated blood.[189] An anticoagulant is used to inactivate the clotting mechanisms so that the sample remains unclotted in the syringe.

Oxylates, ethylenediamine tetraacetic acid (EDTA), and citrates are commonly used as anticoagulants for blood studies. These are not acceptable for blood gas samples because they significantly alter the blood sample.[190, 191]

Heparin is the anticoagulant of choice; however, too much heparin may affect the pH.[192] The pH of sodium heparin is approximately 7.0; P_{CO_2} and P_{O_2} approach room air values.

It can be demonstrated that 0.05 ml sodium heparin (1,000 units/ml or 10 mg/ml) will adequately anticoagulate 1 ml blood; whereas 0.1 ml will not affect pH, P_{CO_2}, or P_{O_2} values of 1 ml blood.[192] When a 5 ml syringe is washed with sodium heparin and then ejected, the dead-space of the syringe will contain approximately 0.15–0.25 ml sodium heparin. Thus, 2–4 ml blood will theoretically contain at least 0.05 ml heparin per 1 ml blood but no more than 0.1 ml heparin per 1 ml blood.

Thus, we recommend the syringe be flushed with sodium heparin (10 mg/ml) and then emptied; this will allow adequate anticoagulation of a 2–4 ml blood sample with assurance that the results will not be altered by the anticoagulant.

Anaerobic Conditions

Room air contains a P_{CO_2} of essentially zero and a P_{O_2} of approximately 150 mm Hg. Air bubbles that mix with a blood sample will result in gas equilibration between the air and the blood. Thus, air bubbles may significantly lower the P_{CO_2} values of the blood sample and cause the P_{O_2} to approach 150 mm Hg. The greater the amount of air mixed with a blood sample, the greater the error.

We recommend that any sample obtained with more than minor air bubbles be discarded. The syringe must be immediately sealed with a cork or a cap after the sample is obtained. The technician must take great care to assure that air does not mix with the sample as it is introduced into the electrode chambers.

Delay in Running the Sample

Blood is living tissue in which oxygen continues to be consumed and carbon dioxide continues to be produced, even after the blood is drawn into a syringe. Table 14–2 shows the approximate rate of change of a sample that is held in the syringe (at 37°C).[193] If the sample is immediately placed in an ice slush, the temperature rapidly falls below 4°C and the P_{CO_2} and pH changes are insignificant over several

TABLE 14–2.—IN VITRO BLOOD GAS CHANGES

	37°C	4°C
pH	0.01/10 min	0.001/10 min
P_{CO_2}	1 mm Hg/10 min	0.1 mm Hg/10 min
P_{O_2}	0.1 vol%/10 min	0.01 vol%/10 min

Approximate changes with time and temperature after the sample is drawn into the syringe. Temperature 37°C assumes that the blood remains at body temperature in the syringe. Temperature 4°C assumes that the sample is properly iced immediately after being drawn.

hours. If the sample is not iced immediately, the changes can be significant.

The white blood cell oxygen consumption is important if the sample is not iced because 0.1 ml oxygen is consumed from 100 ml blood in 10 minutes at body temperature. The effect on oxygen tension depends on the state of hemoglobin saturation.[193] For example, if the P_{O_2} is 400 mm Hg, it will drop to below 250 mm Hg in 1 hour if the sample is not iced. If the sample is immediately placed in an ice slush, the P_{O_2} will be more than 350 mm Hg even after 1 hour. If the P_{O_2} is 50 mm Hg, the loss of 0.1 ml oxygen from 100 ml blood makes a very small change in P_{O_2}, because the primary change is in the hemoglobin saturation (see Fig 9–3).

Reducing the temperature of the blood reduces the metabolic rate of the blood cells. In fact, immediately placing the sample on ice decreases the metabolic rate to such an extent that the sample may undergo little change over several hours. As a general rule, arterial blood samples should be cooled immediately after being drawn; if this is done, a delay of up to 1 hour will have little effect on the results.

Quality Control

Laboratory measurements are only as useful as they are accurate. It may be claimed that inaccurate information is worse than no information, a philosophy that must be adopted by all who are responsible for laboratory values. It is not unusual for very significant clinical decisions to be based largely upon blood gas measurements; for this reason quality control is essential for all blood gas analyzers and the personnel responsible for such machines.

Calibration

The inherent properties of blood gas electrodes (see Chapter 4) make *electronic drift* inevitable. The *potentiometric electrodes* (pH and P_{CO_2}) have a *balance drift;* that is, the low and high calibration points remain on the same angle but shift from baseline (see Chapter 4). This necessitates a one-point balance calibration between blood samples, which is accomplished by introducing a known P_{CO_2} into the Severinghaus electrode and a known pH buffer into the Sanz electrode and adjusting the balance control. The *amperometric electrode* (P_{O_2}) has a slope drift; i.e., the angle of the calibration points changes. This requires a known P_{O_2} to be introduced into the Clark electrode and the slope control adjusted (see Chapter 4).

These calibration procedures assure consistency and accuracy of the electrodes within their limits. However, there is no assurance that the gases and solutions being used as calibration references are correct and consistent. This must be accomplished by external quality control methods.[194-196]

External Controls

These are standards used to test the accuracy and exactness of the known gases and solutions used to calibrate the electrodes.

COMMERCIAL PREPARATIONS. — Presently, there are two commercially available solutions that are reasonably dependable for assuring quality results from the blood gas electrodes. One solution is in a small sealed ampule with pH, P_{CO_2}, and P_{O_2} values predetermined.[197] The other involves reconstitution of a human serum preparation with predetermined pH and P_{CO_2} values.[198] Results obtained from these methods may indicate errors not detectable by calibration methods.

TONOMETRY. — A tonometer is a device that allows equilibration of blood with a known gas.[199, 200] This tonometered blood may be used as a quality control check for P_{CO_2} and P_{O_2}.[201] This system is useful in a high-volume laboratory since it may be more economical on a frequent basis than the commercially available controls.

Minimal Guidelines

We recommend that quality assurance be accomplished *at least* every four hours on every electrode, in addition to complete two-point calibration *at least* every eight hours. One-point calibration should be accomplished before each sample.

The Blood Gas Technician

Nothing can assure quality results better than a well-equipped laboratory (Fig 14–5) staffed by well-trained technicians. Only properly trained individuals can assure that mechanical and technical errors will be corrected immediately. Examples of these problems are: improper temperature settings, contaminated buffers, contaminated gas mixtures, large fluctuations in power line voltages, leaking water baths, membrane ruptures, and numerous others.

Temperature Correction for Blood Gas Values

Most blood gas analyzers report pH, P_{CO_2}, and P_{O_2} data at normal body temperature. In cases of severe hypothermia or hyperthermia,

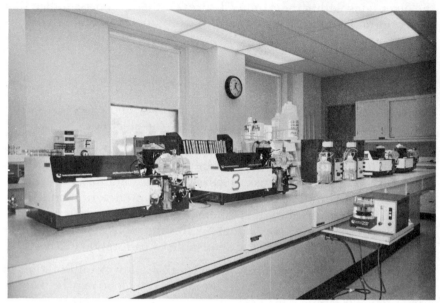

Fig 14–5. – A portion of the Central Blood Gas Laboratory at Northwestern Memorial Hospital.

the blood gas values at 37°C are significantly different from the patient's actual values. Under these conditions the clinician should convert the data at 37°C to the patient's body temperature using the appropriate nomogram.[193, 202]

The clinical application of blood gas measurements is completely dependent upon results that truly reflect the patient status. The appropriate preparation of the sample is essential so that a reliable and accurate laboratory can make the measurements. The following section assumes these conditions—the physician and respiratory care practitioner cannot allow anything less in the care of patients!

SECTION IV

Clinical Application of Blood Gas Measurements

THE PURPOSE of this book is to provide the necessary physiologic and clinical knowledge for the use of blood gas measurements in the supportive care of critically ill patients. Such sophisticated modalities as modern oxygen therapy, bronchial hygiene therapy, and ventilator care, combined with pharmacologic support of the cardiovascular system, maintenance of the fluid and electrolyte balance, and support of renal function, make up a distinct field of clinical endeavor: *critical-care medicine*. A fundamental concern of critical-care medicine is the threat to the basic life process — *gas exchange*. Arterial blood gas analysis not only reflects the state of the basic life process, it also reflects the end result of the supportive modalities.

The following chapters are designed to provide a basis upon which the respiratory care practitioner may *apply* blood gas measurements to the clinical support of critically ill patients. The basic chemistry, physics, physiology, and clinical guidelines previously presented are assumed to be understood; frequent reference to the appropriate previous chapters is provided to aid in the total understanding of the clinical *application* of blood gas measurements.

15 / Oxygen Therapy*

THE APPLICATION OF OXYGEN to ill patients was first attempted over a century and a half ago, and since then it has been shrouded in uncertainty. As late as 1945 there was serious debate in the medical literature as to whether oxygen should have a therapeutic place in medicine. Although blood gas measurements give us the means of properly monitoring oxygen therapy and advances in respiratory therapy have made it possible to administer oxygen properly, few physicians or allied health personnel understand oxygen therapy. Thus, before considering how oxygen therapy affects ventilation and the oxygenation state, it is necessary to clearly state the objectives of oxygen therapy and explain oxygen administration.

Goals of Oxygen Therapy

Before hospitals were air conditioned it was common practice to place a patient in an oxygen tent primarily to cool him on a warm day. Unfortunately, many physicians felt this was the *only* purpose of oxygen administration. Another common practice was to place an oxygen apparatus on the critically ill patient to alleviate his emotional stress. Undoubtedly there is some psychologic value in this, but it is by no means the basic advantage of proper oxygen therapy, which is its physiologic value.

The only direct effect of breathing fractions of inspired oxygen (FI_{O_2}) above 21% is one of the following:

1. The alveolar oxygen tensions may be increased.
2. The ventilatory work necessary to maintain a given alveolar oxygen tension may be decreased.
3. The myocardial work necessary to maintain a given arterial oxygen tension may be decreased.

Through a sound understanding of cardiopulmonary physiology it becomes obvious that there are three clinical goals that can be accomplished with proper oxygen therapy.

Treat hypoxemia. — When arterial hypoxemia is a result of decreased

---

*Portions of this chapter originally appeared in Shapiro, B. A., Harrison, R. A., and Trout, C. A.: *Clinical Application of Respiratory Care* (Chicago: Year Book Medical Publishers, Inc., 1975).

alveolar oxygen tensions, that hypoxemia may be dramatically improved by increasing the inspired oxygen fractions.

Decrease the work of breathing. — Increased ventilatory work is a common response to hypoxemia and/or hypoxia. Enriched inspired oxygen atmospheres may allow a more normal alveolar gas exchange to maintain adequate alveolar oxygen levels. The result is a decreased need for total ventilation, which means a decreased work of breathing at no expense to the oxygenation status.

Decrease myocardial work. — The cardiovascular system is a primary mechanism for compensation of hypoxemia and/or hypoxia (see Chapter 9). Oxygen therapy can effectively support many disease states by decreasing or preventing the demand for increased myocardial work.

Administration of Oxygen

Fraction of Inspired Oxygen

Having established clear clinical goals, the evaluation of the adequacy and effectiveness of oxygen therapy is a matter of clinical examination and blood gas measurement — as long as the administration of oxygen is consistent and predictable! This necessitates a knowledge of oxygen devices, techniques, and inspired oxygen fractions.

Normal variances in the distribution of ventilation and pulmonary blood flow make the measurement of alveolar oxygen concentrations impractical and complex. Significant variation in oxygen concentration may occur throughout the inspiratory cycle; where and when to make the measurement is not universally agreed upon. Attempts at sampling tracheal air have been limited because of the slow electrode response time of available equipment.[203, 204] Recent technical advances have made this measurement more practical, but the clinical application of an "invasive" technique remains difficult to justify for routine use. The necessity exists for having a measurement that can be easily, practically, and consistently used in the clinical setting to reflect inspired oxygen concentrations. Such a measurement might be the percent (fraction) of inspired gas that is oxygen (FI_{O_2}).

Clinical definition of FI_{O_2}. — Since the final judgment of the adequacy of oxygen therapy is made by blood gas analysis and clinical examination, the major requisites of oxygen administration are *consistency* and *control*. Logic dictates that the most reasonable approach is to define the FI_{O_2} as the *measurable* or *calculable* concentration of oxygen delivered to the patient; i.e., if a tidal volume of 500 ml is composed of 250 ml oxygen, the FI_{O_2} will be considered 50%. In other words, we will not be concerned with how the gases are distributed throughout the tracheobronchial tree and the lung parenchyma; the concern will be solely with the fact that 50% of the entire inspired atmosphere is oxygen. This provides us with a consistent, practical, and understandable terminology that is easily applied to any method of oxygen therapy. With this arbitrary definition accepted, reliable oxygen therapy becomes a matter of methodology and thorough understanding of oxygen delivery systems.

Gas Delivery Systems

The advent of anesthetic gases and their clinical administration necessitated the development of gas delivery systems to meet various needs. The past century has seen a myriad of techniques developed for delivering controlled gas concentrations.[205] All these techniques fall into one of two categories: non-rebreathing and rebreathing systems.

NON-REBREATHING SYSTEMS (FIG 15–1).—A non-rebreathing system is designed so that exhaled gases have minimal contact with inspiratory gases. In most cases, this is simply a matter of venting the exhaled gases to the atmosphere via one-way valves. A primary advantage to

Fig 15–1.—A model non-rebreathing system. The gas source must supply a volume at least equal to the patient's minute ventilation. A reservoir bag serves to make gas available to meet peak flow requirements. A one-way valve system (at points *a*) assures that the patient will inhale only fresh gas and exhale only to the room atmosphere. A one-way valve (*b*) will allow room air to supply a portion of the inspiratory volume if the gas source and reservoir prove inadequate. (From Shapiro, B. A., Harrison, R. A., and Trout, C. A.: *Clinical Application of Respiratory Care* [Chicago: Year Book Medical Publishers, Inc., 1975].)

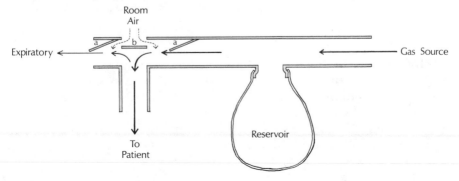

non-rebreathing systems is that exhaled carbon dioxide does not have to be dealt with in the inspiratory gas system. However, a gas flow sufficient to meet the requirements of the minute volume and peak flow rate must be supplied. This is usually accomplished by an inspiratory reservoir which allows an additional amount of gas to be available during the transient times when inspiratory demands are beyond the capabilities of the uniform flow rates delivered by the apparatus.

To better meet this problem of sufficient gas delivery, non-rebreathing systems have been developed in which a one-way valve allows room air to enter if the system itself is not adequate to meet the ventilatory demands. In this way, adequate minute volume and peak inspiratory flow volume are assured. This is accomplished at the expense of diluting the initially delivered gas concentrations with room air.

A non-rebreathing system in which the minute volume, flow rates, and reservoir system are adequate to meet the total ventilatory needs of the patient is called a *high-flow system*. Whenever room air must enter the system to meet total gas requirements, the system is considered a *low-flow system*. In other words, *low-flow non-rebreathing systems do not allow inspired gas mixtures to be determined precisely.*

REBREATHING SYSTEMS. — A rebreathing system is one in which a reservoir exists on the expiratory line and a carbon dioxide absorber is present so that the exhaled air minus the CO_2 can re-enter the inspiratory system. Rebreathing systems gained popularity in anesthesia because of their potential for conserving expensive anesthetic gases and because many anesthetic gases are explosive.

During induction of anesthesia, the rebreathing system is often used as a high-flow, non-rebreathing system. By preventing exhaled gases from diluting fresh inspired gas, the concentration of anesthetic gases delivered to the patient is kept constant. In other words, anesthesiology has long recognized that high-flow, non-rebreathing systems are most desirable for precise control of inspired gas mixtures.[206]

Oxygen Delivery Systems

Modern oxygen therapy is properly administered by *non-rebreathing systems* because: (1) oxygen is a nonexplosive agent; (2) the expense is not prohibitive; and (3) rebreathing CO_2 is easily avoided. Since we are dealing with oxygen delivery and non-rebreathing systems, we may think in terms of high-flow and low-flow systems.

The *high-flow system* is defined as one in which the gas flow of the apparatus is sufficient to meet all inspiratory requirements. A *low-flow system* is one in which the gas flow of the apparatus is *in*sufficient to meet all inspiratory requirements. Thus, room air must be used to provide part of the inspired atmosphere.

Most of the confusion surrounding oxygen therapy results from referring to the *technique* rather than to the *device*. Low-*concentration* oxygen techniques were unfortunately described in terms of oxygen *flow rate* through a nasal cannula. This "low-flow oxygen administration" has led much of the medical world to believe that low flow is synonymous with low concentration. *Since it is the fraction of inspired oxygen that is important, oxygen flow should be considered only in relation to the total gas flow.* The concentration of oxygen delivered by any oxygen flow rate is determined solely by the apparatus and patient.

Fig 15–2.—A Venturi device providing high total gas flow at fixed FI_{O_2}. Pressurized oxygen is forced through a narrow orifice; Bernoulli's principle determines the amount of room air entrained (see text). A Venturi mask is depicted; however, the Venturi mechanism is found in almost all high-flow oxygen delivery systems. (From Shapiro, B. A., Harrison, R. A., and Trout, C. A.: *Clinical Application of Respiratory Care* [Chicago: Year Book Medical Publishers, 1975].)

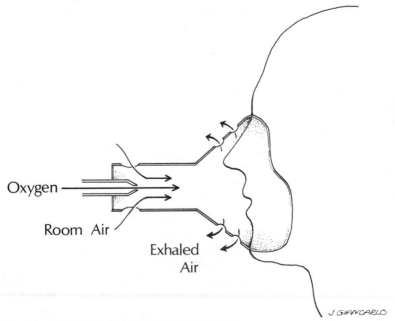

Oxygen

Room Air

Exhaled
Air

J GIANCARLO

TABLE 15-1.—APPROXIMATE AIR ENTRAINMENT RATIO

OXYGEN CONCENTRATION (%)	AIR°/100% O_2
24	25/1
28	10/1
34	5/1
40	3/1
60	1/1
70	0.6/1

Examples:
  a. 40% Venturi device—10 L/min O_2 flow will produce a total gas flow of approximately 40 L/min.
  b. 28% Venturi device—4 L/min O_2 flow will produce a total gas flow of approximately 44 L/min.
  °Room air is assumed to be 20.9% oxygen.

HIGH-FLOW OXYGEN SYSTEMS. — A high-flow oxygen system is one in which the flow rate and reservoir capacity are adequate to provide the total inspired atmosphere. In other words, the patient is breathing only the gas that is supplied by the apparatus. The characteristics of a high-flow oxygen delivery system are distinct from the *concentration* of oxygen provided; both high and low oxygen concentrations may be administered by high-flow systems.

Most high-flow oxygen delivery systems use a *Venturi device* (Fig 15–2), i.e., a system using the Bernoulli principle to "entrain" room air in static proportion to oxygen flows (Table 15–1). Such a device provides high total gas flows of fixed FI_{O_2}. The Bernoulli principle states that the lateral pressure of a gas decreases as its velocity of flow increases. Therefore, an oxygen flow through a constricted orifice, because of its great increase in velocity of flow, can create a "subatmospheric" pressure just after leaving the orifice. This subatmospheric pressure "entrains" room air. By varying the orifice size and oxygen flow, the FI_{O_2} may be varied.

High-flow systems can provide concentrations of 24–100% oxygen. There are *Venturi masks* available that provide 24–40% oxygen in addition to nebulizers utilizing the Venturi principle that can provide 30–100% oxygen concentrations. Numerous valves and appliances are available to provide varying FI_{O_2}s through high-flow systems.

High-flow systems have two major advantages: (1) because consistent FI_{O_2}s are provided as long as the system is properly applied, changes in the patient's ventilatory pattern do not affect the FI_{O_2}; and (2) since the entire inspired atmosphere is provided, the temperature and humidity of the gas may be controlled.

FI_{O_2} can be directly measured in a high-flow system with an oxygen analyzer. Numerous analyzers are commercially available and most are reliable and accurate when properly used and maintained. The fact that oxygen concentration can be *measured* in a high-flow system is a significant advantage for critically ill patients. If not for the disadvantages of economics and patient comfort, high-flow systems would certainly be the method of choice for all oxygen therapy.

LOW-FLOW OXYGEN SYSTEMS. — The low-flow system does not provide sufficient gas to supply the entire inspired atmosphere; therefore, part of the tidal volume must be supplied by breathing room air. Any concentration of oxygen from 21% to 90+% can be provided by such a system. The variables controlling FI_{O_2} are: (1) the capacity of the available oxygen reservoir; (2) the oxygen flow (L/min); and (3) the patient's ventilatory pattern. These systems are used because of tradition, familiarity, patient comfort, economics, and availability — *not* because of accuracy or dependability.

In principle, low-flow systems depend primarily upon the existence of a *reservoir* of oxygen and its dilution with room air. To demonstrate the use of low-flow systems, let us consider a "normal" person with a "normal" ventilatory pattern:

Tidal volume (V_T)	500 ml
Ventilatory rate (RR)	20/min
Inspiratory time	1 sec
Expiratory time	2 sec
Anatomic reservoir	50 ml

The anatomic reservoir is composed of the nose, the nasopharynx, and the oropharynx (Fig 15–3). We will assume that the volume of the anatomic reservoir is one third of the anatomic deadspace; therefore, $1/3 \times 150$ ml = 50 ml.

A nasal cannula with an oxygen flow of 6 L/min (100 ml/sec) is placed on this patient. We can safely assume that most of the expired flow occurs during the first 1.5 sec (75%) of the expiratory time; i.e., the last 0.5 sec of expiration has negligible expired gas flow. This allows the anatomic reservoir to fill completely with 100% oxygen because the flow rate is 50 ml/0.5 sec (100 ml/sec).

Assuming all oxygen supplied by the cannula and contained in the anatomic reservoir is inspired by the patient, the next 500 ml tidal volume, which takes 1 sec, is composed of:

50 ml of 100% oxygen from the anatomic reservoir.

100 ml of 100% oxygen supplied by the cannula flow rate.

350 ml of 20% oxygen (room air); thus, 0.20×350 ml = 70 ml oxygen.

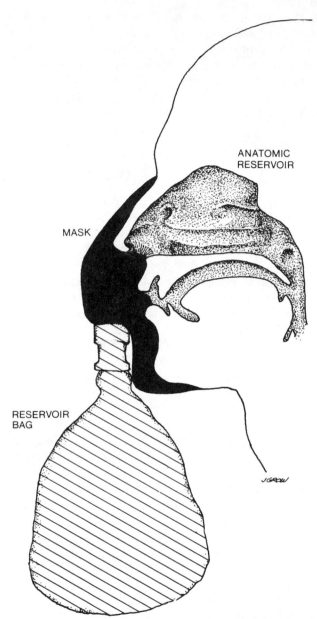

Fig 15–3.—Reservoirs in low-flow oxygen therapy. The *anatomic reservoir* consists of the nose, the nasopharynx, and the oropharynx. This reservoir is estimated to be approximately one third of the anatomic deadspace. The *appliance reservoir* consists of (1) the mask – 100 to 200 ml volume, depending on the appliance; and (2) the reservoir bag – 600 to 1,000 ml added volume.

The 500 ml of inspired gas contain 220 ml of 100% oxygen: 50 ml + 100 ml + 70ml = 220 ml. We calculate:

$$\frac{220 \text{ ml oxygen}}{500 \text{ ml}} = 44\% \text{ oxygen}$$

This means that a patient with an "ideal ventilatory pattern" who receives 6 L/min of oxygen flow by nasal cannula is receiving an FI_{O_2} of 44%.

If we compute for this person all flows from 1 L to 6 L by nasal cannula or catheter, we see that for every liter-per-minute change in flow rate there is approximately a 4% change in the inspired oxygen fraction (Table 15–2, A).

For practical application, we must have some guidelines for "estimating" the FI_{O_2} that a given low-flow apparatus with a given oxygen flow will deliver to a patient. It is essential to understand that *the FI_{O_2} in a low-flow system varies tremendously with changes in tidal volume and ventilatory pattern.*

Let us consider the same patient with his tidal volume reduced by half: 250 ml instead of 500 ml. The quantities now are:

50 ml of 100% oxygen from the anatomic reservoir.
100 ml of 100% oxygen determined by the cannula flow rate.
100 ml of 20% oxygen (room air).

TABLE 15–2.—GUIDELINES FOR ESTIMATING FI_{O_2} WITH LOW-FLOW OXYGEN DEVICES

100% O_2 FLOW RATE (L)	$FI_{O_2}(\%)$
A. Nasal cannula or catheter:	
1	24
2	28
3	32
4	36
5	40
6	44
B. Oxygen mask:	
5–6	40
6–7	50
7–8	60
C. Mask with reservoir bag:	
6	60
7	70
8	80
9	90
10	99+

Note: Normal ventilatory pattern is assumed.

Thus, the 250 ml of inspired gas contains 170 ml of 100% oxygen: 50 ml + 100 ml + 20 ml = 170 ml. We calculate:

$$\frac{170 \text{ ml oxygen}}{250 \text{ ml}} = 68\% \text{ oxygen}$$

In a low-flow system, the larger the tidal volume, the lower the FI_{O_2}; or the smaller the tidal volume, the higher the FI_{O_2}.

A low-flow system delivers consistent oxygen concentrations as long as the ventilatory pattern is unchanged. However, it is erroneous to assume *that a nasal cannula guarantees low-concentration oxygen.* Obviously, a 1 or 2 L oxygen flow in a patient breathing shallowly can deliver much higher oxygen concentrations than one would be led to believe.

A nasal cannula can be used as long as the nasal passages are patent, since mouth breathing does not affect FI_{O_2}. The airflow in the oropharynx creates a Bernoulli effect in the nasopharynx and air is inspired through the nose. Remember, the *nasal passages must be patent.*

A nasal cannula or catheter with more than a 6 L flow does little to increase inspired oxygen concentrations, primarily because the anatomic reservoir is filled. Thus, in order to provide a higher FI_{O_2} with a low-flow system, one has to increase the size of the oxygen reservoir. This is accomplished by placing a mask over the nose and mouth, thus increasing the volume of the potential oxygen reservoir (see Fig 15–3). This type of apparatus gives the inspired oxygen concentration shown in Table 15–2, B, as long as the ventilatory pattern is normal.

An oxygen mask should never be run at less than a 5 L flow; otherwise, exhaled air accumulating in the mask reservoir might be rebreathed. Above 5 L/min, most of the exhaled air will be flushed from the mask. Above an 8 L flow there is little increase in the inspired oxygen concentration because the reservoir is filled. Of course, changes in ventilatory pattern are as important in affecting the inspired oxygen concentrations as they are with the cannula and the catheter.

To deliver more than 60% oxygen by a low-flow system, one must again increase the oxygen reservoir (see Fig 15–3). This is accomplished by attaching a reservoir bag to the mask (see Table 15–2, C). Without a one-way valve between the bag and mask, this apparatus is called a *partial rebreathing mask.* This bag is neither a carbon dioxide reservoir nor a rebreathing bag. It is meant to be an *oxygen reservoir;* therefore, the bag must never be totally collapsed during inspiration. The very early exhaled air (the first one third of exhalation) will go back into the bag. This is deadspace air from the mouth and the trachea and contains little carbon dioxide. Again, it must be remembered that this is a low-flow system, in which the inspired oxygen concentrations vary according to the ventilatory pattern. At flow rates from $6-10$ L/min, a close-fitting mask with reservoir bag gives approximately $60-90+\%$ oxygen.

SUMMARY. — With these basic guidelines for oxygen administration in mind, one can readily provide a patient with a consistent and predictable oxygen concentration. Increasing or decreasing the inspired oxygen concentrations within reasonably predictable limits is possible and, most important, we can deliver a *consistent* oxygen concentration. A patient with a shallow, deep, or irregular ventilatory pattern should receive oxygen therapy from a high-flow system rather than from a low-flow system.[11] It must be clearly understood that even though the term *low-flow oxygen* is generally considered to mean low-concentration oxygen, this may not be the case. The ventilatory pattern must be assessed! *As long as oxygen administration is consistent and predictable, clinical observation plus blood gas measurement will assure proper oxygen therapy.*

Blood Gas Abnormalities and Oxygen Therapy

Hypoxemia

As outlined in chapter 9, hypoxemia may be due to decreased alveolar oxygen tension (including venous admixture), increased absolute shunting, or decreased central venous oxygen content. *Only hypoxemia due to a decreased* $P_{A_{O_2}}$ *will respond dramatically to oxygen therapy.* This should be obvious, because the prime purpose of breathing increased oxygen atmospheres is to increase the alveolar oxygen tension. In other words, hypoxemia responds dramatically to oxygen therapy when that hypoxemia is the result of hypoventilation, oxygen diffusion impedance, or venous admixture (shunt effect).

The absolute physiologic shunt is the measurement of anatomic and capillary shunts, i.e., those instances in which there is no exchange of blood with alveolar air. With absolute shunting the right ventricular blood is deposited into the left ventricle without respiring — without any gas exchange. With venous admixture (shunt effect) some gas exchange takes place, but perfusion exceeds ventilation (see Chapter 9).

Figure $15-4$ demonstrates how the absolute shunt may be theoretically separated from venous admixture by having the patient breathe 100% oxygen for at least 15 minutes. By this "denitrogenation" pro-

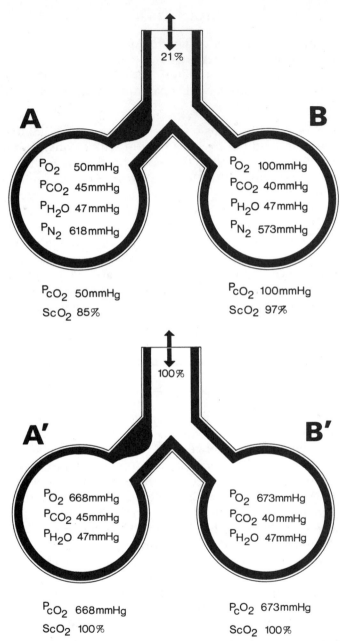

Fig 15–4.—Separating the absolute shunt from venous admixture by breathing 100% oxygen for 15 minutes. Alveoli **A** and **B** represent room air breathing; alveoli **A′** and **B′** represent alveolar gases following denitrogenation. Note that any meaningful PA_{O_2} difference is ablated after denitrogenation.

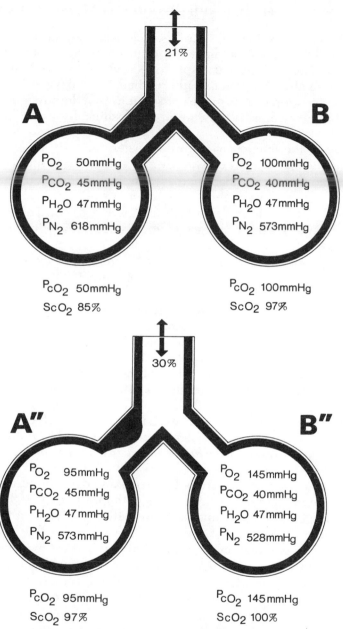

Fig 15–5. — Venous admixture and 30%FI_{O_2}. Alveoli **A** and **B** represent room air breathing. Alveoli **A″** and **B″** represent alveolar gases following 30% oxygen administration for 15 minutes. The aveolar oxygen tension has been increased to the point where Pc_{O_2} is 95 mm Hg and Sc_{O_2} is 97%. The venous admixture hypoxemia is gone. This is the principle behind low-concentration Oxygen therapy and ventilation perfusion inequality.

cess the alveolar oxygen tensions become nearly equal, as seen in alveoli A' and B' — venous admixture (perfusion in excess of ventilation) has been ablated. Clinical attempts to measure absolute shunt used to be measured after the patient had breathed 100% oxygen for 15 minutes. A better appreciation of the consequences of denitrogenation has changed the concepts as they are applied clinically (see Chapters 9 and 19).[11]

Increasing the fraction of inspired oxygen (FI_{O_2}) by 10% increases the ideal alveolar oxygen tension by approximately 45 mm Hg.[207] We may assume that these small increases in inspired oxygen concentration have a great effect on the end pulmonary capillary oxygen tension (Pc_{O_2}) of alveoli that have venous admixture (Fig 15–5). The increased capillary oxygen tension causes a significant increase in the oxygen content.

Thus, *oxygen therapy produces a profound compensatory effect for the arterial hypoxemia due to venous admixture.*[208] This explains why hypoxemia due to ventilation/perfusion inequality is so responsive to the administration of 24–40% inspired oxygen; e.g., in chronic obstructive pulmonary disease or retained secretions.

On the other hand, hypoxemia due to absolute shunting is not nearly as responsive to increased inspired oxygen concentrations.[209] Alveolar oxygen tensions are usually near normal or higher in the areas of the lung that are being ventilated. Little additional oxygen can be added to the blood by increasing these alveolar oxygen tensions. The blood that is shunting does not exchange with the alveolar air and therefore is unaffected by alveolar oxygen tensions. *The primary compensatory mechanism for the hypoxemia caused by absolute shunting is an increase in cardiac output.*

In summary, the response of a hypoxemia to oxygen therapy is primarily dependent upon the underlying pathophysiology. If the hypoxemia is due to absolute shunting, there will be little effect from oxygen therapy; if a significant part of the hypoxemia is due to uneven distribution of ventilation (venous admixture), there will be a profound response to oxygen therapy. Blood gas analysis is essential to the monitoring of oxygen therapy. *Proper interpretation of arterial blood gases is the cornerstone of supportive oxygen therapy.*

Alveolar Hyperventilation

Alveolar hyperventilation (see Chapter 8) may have three physiologic origins: (1) hypoxemia, (2) response to metabolic acidosis, or (3) central nervous system response. It is unusual to find significant hypoxemia when alveolar hyperventilation is due to the second or third cause. Therefore it is a reasonable assumption that *whenever alveolar hyperventilation with moderate or severe hypoxemia is present, the alveolar hyperventilation is probably secondary to the hypoxemic state.*

When alveolar hyperventilation is the result of arterial hypoxemia, both the cardiovascular and the pulmonary systems are working harder to maintain that arterial oxygen tension at which the peripheral chemoreceptors (see Chapter 9) are minimally stimulated.[210] When an increased oxygen atmosphere is breathed, the alveolar oxygen tensions will most likely be increased. *The increased $P_{A_{O_2}}$ means that the heart and the ventilatory muscles can do less work and still maintain the arterial oxygen tension at the level that preceded oxygen therapy.* The organism will not preferentially increase the arterial oxygen tension level if ventilatory work is great or if myocardial work is significantly increased. In essence, then, *the patient manifesting alveolar hyperventilation secondary to hypoxemia will preferentially decrease ventilatory and myocardial work in response to oxygen therapy, rather than increase arterial oxygen tensions to nonhypoxemic levels.*

Below are the blood gas measurements and the vital signs of a 35-year-old man with bilateral pneumonia (BP = blood pressure, P = pulse, and RR = respiratory rate):

pH	7.52	BP	150/100
P_{CO_2}	28 mm Hg	P	130/min
P_{O_2}	60 mm Hg	RR	32/min
		VT	500 ml
		MV	16 L

Physical examination showed the patient to be sweating, anxious, and complaining of difficulty in breathing. Note the hypertension, tachycardia, and tachypnea. His blood gases reveal an acute alveolar hyperventilation with mild to moderate arterial hypoxemia.

An oxygen mask that delivered approximately 50% oxygen was placed and 30 minutes later the patient was comfortable and had no subjective complaints. Repeat studies revealed:

pH	7.45	BP	120/80
P_{CO_2}	35 mm Hg	P	100/min
P_{O_2}	70 mm Hg	RR	22/min
		VT	450 ml
		MV	9.9 L

His blood pressure was normal, and the tachycardia and tachypnea were significantly decreased. Arterial blood gas analysis revealed a marked decrease in alveolar ventilation and an increase in arterial oxygen tension. The most striking changes due to oxygen therapy were the decreases in ventilatory and myocardial work.

The need for oxygen therapy would not be fully appreciated if one were to judge the effect of oxygen therapy by the arterial oxygen tension alone. However, the value of oxygen therapy is obvious when one understands that the original purpose of delivering oxygen to this patient was to support the cardiovascular and ventilatory systems by decreasing their work. In other words, the oxygen therapy was not used primarily to treat the hypoxemia; rather, it was used to decrease the work of breathing and the myocardial work while maintaining a satisfactory oxygenation status.

Another example is a 55-year-old man admitted to the coronary care unit with a diagnosis of inferior wall infarct. He complained of severe chest pain, and his ECG showed ventricular arrhythmia. His blood gases were interpreted as being within an acceptable ventilatory range with a moderate hypoxemia:

pH	7.42	BP	140/90
P_{CO_2}	33 mm Hg	P	130/min, irregular
P_{O_2}	55 mm Hg	RR	25/min

Administration of 40% oxygen improved the alveolar ventilation and improved the hypoxemia somewhat:

pH	7.40	BP	120/80
P_{CO_2}	37 mm Hg	P	110/min, regular
P_{O_2}	60 mm Hg	RR	20/min

Note that the pulse became regular and decreased to 110/min, tachypnea was reduced, and the patient had far less chest pain. In this case, myocardial oxygenation was probably improved by decreasing the myocardial work that resulted from the hypoxemia. The reader must not get the impression that oxygen is an anti-arrhythmic drug; this example is meant to emphasize the importance of oxygen therapy for purposes other than dramatically increasing the arterial P_{O_2}.

Acute Ventilatory Failure

When the body is suddenly deprived of adequate alveolar ventilation, acidemia and hypoxemia inevitably follow. This combination rapidly leads to tissue hypoxia. *High arterial carbon dioxide tension with acidemia is defined as acute ventilatory failure.* The severity is judged on the degree of acidemia and the clinical situation. Until proven otherwise, acute ventilatory failure is a medical emergency! The ventilatory system must be immediately supported unless the precipitating cause can be rapidly reversed. Proper mechanical support of ventilation will usually reestablish normal alveolar ventilation, and this should reverse the acidemia and hypoxemia. *Oxygen therapy is secondary in the support of acute ventilatory failure, because oxygen therapy alone cannot improve the ventilatory status in this circumstance.*

Chronic Ventilatory Failure and Oxygen Therapy

This condition is usually secondary to chronic obstructive pulmonary disease. The patient has adjusted to his ventilatory failure and is not in acute distress. As shown in Figure 8-1, this is the classic "respiratory failure" patient: the arterial carbon dioxide tension is greater than 50 mm Hg and the arterial oxygen tension is less than 50 mm Hg. The disease has resulted in high airway resistance, deadspace, and shunting, which together have resulted in a high oxygen cost of breathing. The great work of breathing has forced the patient to settle for inadequate alveolar ventilation and low arterial oxygen tension (see Chapter 8). He depends greatly upon the heart's ability to maintain an adequate cardiac output, so he has little cardiopulmonary reserve to meet physiologic stress. His drive to breathe is primarily from chemoreceptor stimulation.[211]

The typical patient is a 70-year-old man with a diagnosis of chronic obstructive pulmonary disease. At rest his vital signs and blood gases are:

pH	7.43	BP	160/120
P_{CO_2}	65 mm Hg	P	110/min
P_{O_2}	43 mm Hg	RR	30/min
		V_T	300 ml
		MV	9L

It should be noted that the patient has a pH greater than 7.40. This is typical and is believed to be due to water and chloride ion shifts between intracellular and extracellular spaces, occurring as part of the metabolic compensation for the respiratory acidemia.[212]

It must be remembered that this patient breathes primarily in response to chemoreceptor stimuli and *only* hard enough to retain his baseline hypoxemic state. Administering 40% oxygen to this patient will result in a *profound* decrease in the demand for ventilation; that is, the increased *alveolar* oxygen tension allows the usual arterial oxygen tension to be maintained at even less alveolar ventilation than before the oxygen was administered. *The organism will elect to breathe less hard rather than increase the Pa_{O_2}.* This results in an acute *decrease* in alveolar ventilation (increased Pa_{CO_2}) and acidemia.

The vital signs and blood gases of this patient on 40% oxygen may be:

pH	7.20	BP	200/40
PCO^2	90 mm Hg	P	140/min
PO_2	60 mm Hg	RR	45/min, shallow
		VT	200 ml
		MV	9L

Oxygen therapy has produced an acute ventilatory failure! This acute decrease in alveolar ventilation is superimposed on the chronic ventilatory failure. Despite improved arterial oxygen tensions, the acute acidemia and general central nervous system obtundation now threaten tissue oxygenation to a greater degree than the pre-existing hypoxemia.

The primary effect of oxygen therapy in patients with chronic ventilatory failure is the change in ventilatory status. This is not true in acute ventilatory failure or in other conditions where the drive to breathe is *not* chemoreceptor stimulation from hypoxemia.

Much confusion and misinformation exist concerning the application of low concentrations of oxygen to support "respiratory failure." A clear understanding of the pathophysiology and pathogenesis of chronic ventilatory failure makes the clinical application of oxygen predictable and understandable in its supportive role (see Chapter 8). Remember, oxygen therapy is never a cure! Proper application of oxygen will, one hopes, support the patient's cardiopulmonary system by improving the ventilatory status. This will improve the oxygenation status while other measures are instituted to reverse the cause of the acute process.

Acute Ventilatory Failure Superimposed on Chronic Ventilatory Failure: The "Low-Concentration Oxygen" Technique

The typical patient for the "low-concentration oxygen" technique is the "chronic lunger." He suffers from chronic ventilatory failure and has acquired an acute disease such as infectious pneumonia. In response to an acute shunt-producing disease, he attempts to increase his ventilatory and myocardial work to maintain the baseline Pa_{O_2}. However, he finds it detrimental to increase ventilatory work, because in doing so he consumes more oxygen than is gained with increased alveolar ventilation (see Chapter 8). And so, in an attempt to meet the hypoxemic challenge of the increased shunt, he begins to breathe *less*. On room air his blood gases and vital signs might be:

pH	7.25	BP	200/140
P_{CO_2}	90 mm Hg	P	140/min
P_{O_2}	30 mm Hg	RR	45/min, labored
		V_T	200 ml
		MV	9 L

Tissue hypoxia ensues because of the combination of hypoxemia and acidemia, and in response the patient breathes less and less. This physiologic vicious cycle leads to death. If one were to judge the severity of ventilatory failure on Pa_{CO_2} alone, this patient would appear to be *in extremis*. However, the pH is *not* severely acidemic, which means the *acute* change in alveolar ventilation has not been as great as the 90 mm Hg Pa_{CO_2} would lead one to believe. *The severity of acute ventilatory failure is judged on the severity of acidemia.*

The patient has a great deal of venous admixture (shunt effect) because of his chronic obstructive pulmonary disease. Therefore, very small increases in inspired oxygen concentration will have profound effects on arterial oxygenation. Increased *alveolar* oxygen tensions will allow this patient to meet the *acute* hypoxemic challenge without the demand for changing ventilation; that is, he will be able to resume the baseline hypoventilatory state and still maintain his baseline hypoxemic state.

Thirty minutes after 24% oxygen, the readings might be:

pH	7.30	BP	200/140
P_{CO_2}	80 mm Hg	P	130/min
P_{O_2}	40 mm Hg	RR	40/min, labored

The paradox is that this patient's response to oxygen is to increase alveolar ventilation, maintaining arterial oxygen tensions at the highest possible level. *The oxygen therapy has allowed the patient to increase alveolar ventilation back to his baseline level without sacrificing tissue oxygenation.* This leads to decreases in the acidemia and in the tissue hypoxia. The increased tissue oxygenation state allows even better alveolar ventilation, and by increasing the $F_{I_{O_2}}$ to 28%, the following measurements are obtained after several hours:

pH	7.35	BP	170/120
P_{CO_2}	70 mm Hg	P	120/min
P_{O_2}	45 mm Hg	RR	35/min

The oxygen therapy has manipulated the ventilatory status so that the acute acidemia, and therefore the acute tissue hypoxia, are gone. In addition, the improved arterial P_{O_2} and pH have decreased pulmonary artery pressures and thereby improved right heart function. This allows the patient to maintain a good cardiopulmonary status for the next 24–36 hours, while the acute infectious pneumonia is being treated.

Proper oxygen therapy allows this patient to maintain his normal tissue oxygenation state *without* demands to increase his ventilatory work. He is thus able to tolerate the acute increase in shunting without requiring ventilator support. If this patient's response to low concentrations of oxygen had not been an improvement in alveolar ventilation and pH, it might have been necessary to institute ventilatory support. Blood gas analysis makes this response obvious within several hours of the patient's presenting with his acute problem, and the decision of whether or not mechanical support of ventilation will be needed is usually quite evident after this time.

High-flow oxygen delivery systems should be used when feasible, because these patients often have irregular and shallow breathing patterns.

Acute Alveolar Hyperventilation Superimposed on Chronic Ventilatory Failure

Not all chronic ventilatory failure patients with an acute shunting disease present as an acute ventilatory failure superimposed on a chronic ventilatory failure. Some patients possess the strength to increase alveolar ventilation and present as acute alveolar hyperventilation superimposed on a chronic ventilatory failure, as the following blood gas measurements show:

pH	7.52
P_{CO_2}	55 mm Hg
P_{O_2}	45 mm Hg

These measurements would be initially interpreted as partially compensated metabolic alkalosis *with hypoxemia* (see Chapter 13). Whenever such an interpretation is made, one must be alert to the possibility that this may be acute alveolar hyperventilation superimposed on a chronic ventilatory failure.

The chronic ventilatory failure patient who responds to an acute disease by increasing alveolar ventilation responds to supportive oxygen therapy in the same way as any patient with an alveolar hyperventilation secondary to hypoxemia. Thus, 24% oxygen in this patient results in an increase in alveolar oxygen tension and a decrease in alveolar ventilation to the baseline state:

pH	7.45
P_{CO_2}	65 mm Hg
P_{O_2}	50 mm Hg

Great care must be taken to prevent the administration of too much oxygen.

Oxygen Toxicity

The fact that high concentrations (greater than 50–60%) of oxygen administered for long periods (3 days to weeks) may cause acute pulmonary toxicity is well documented.[213] *However, it is essential to keep in mind the relative danger of hypoxia and hyperoxia.* The pathophysiology of hypoxia in the critically ill patient has been aggressively treated for only two decades. In that time, numerous therapeutic manipulations, including oxygen therapy, have become normal practice. In the application of these treatment techniques, oxygen has often been abused and there is little room for disagreement that oxygen toxicity is a real iatrogenic (doctor-induced) disease. However, an overreaction to the dangers associated with oxygen supplementation has led to an extremely hazardous circumstance — poorly informed clinicians withholding essential oxygen therapy from hypoxic or hypoxemic patients. *To allow a patient to be exposed to dangerous levels of hypoxia for fear of developing oxygen toxicity is intolerable!* It is essential to remember that hypoxia is common and that the damage it causes is rapid and severe. On the other hand, pulmonary injury from oxygen is uncommon and its development is relatively slow.

Careful consideration of all the evidence, along with sound clinical principles, leads us to make three generalizations concerning oxygen therapy and oxygen toxicity.

1. Inspired oxygen tensions below 50% at 1 atmosphere rarely produce acute pulmonary oxygen toxicity — even with prolonged exposures. Under normobaric conditions there should be no hesitation

in providing appropriate low-concentration oxygen (less than 50%) for supportive therapy of the cardiopulmonary system. Even in conjunction with appropriately administered intermittent positive-pressure ventilation, low-concentration oxygen rarely produces pulmonary toxicity.

2. Pulmonary oxygen toxicity in man has *not* been demonstrated from breathing 100% oxygen for 24 hours or less. Therefore, oxygen toxicity should not be a consideration intraoperatively, in resuscitation, or in transport situations. *Pure oxygen has no contraindication for brief periods in emergency situations!* However, absorption atelectasis must be kept in mind as a potential problem since this can occur within 30 minutes. The lowest possible $F_{I_{O_2}}$ should be administered as early as feasible in the clinical course.

3. Patients with pre-existing pulmonary disease are no more prone to develop acute pulmonary oxygen toxicity than patients with normal lungs. However, pre-existing pulmonary disease is more susceptible to absorption atelectasis. Our clinical concern of acute pulmonary oxygen toxicity must not differ between the pre-existing nondiseased and diseased lung. *The general principle of minimal oxygen administration consistent with adequate cardiopulmonary homeostasis always holds true!*

High $F_{I_{O_2}}$s are most commonly administered to patients with primary cardiopulmonary disease. Therefore, although the pre-existing pulmonary diseased patient has no *inherent* increased risk of acute pulmonary oxygen toxicity, he is the patient who will most likely receive high oxygen concentrations. All measures possible must be instituted to allow minimal $F_{I_{O_2}}$s for maintenance of adequate oxygenation. Such measures include optimal ventilatory patterns, fluid restriction, maintenance of electrolyte and acid-base balance, and the institution of positive end-expiratory pressure (PEEP) where indicated. Of course, basic modalities of bronchial hygiene to improve distribution of ventilation and decreased work of breathing are essential.

The avoidance of excessively high inspired oxygen concentrations is a common issue in critical-care units. One must realize that appropriate tissue oxygenation is essential to the maintenance of life, especially in patients with multi-organ systems disease. There can be no dogmatic guidelines concerning appropriate degrees of arterial oxygenation to assure tissue oxygenation. This must always be a clinical decision based on thorough knowledge of cardiopulmonary homeostasis, careful monitoring, and physical examination.

Arterial blood gas measurement is essential for the appropriate administration of oxygen therapy!!

16 / Shunt and Deadspace Disease

THE CARDIOPULMONARY homeostatic schema (see Fig 5–1) is an exquisite balance of gas exchange between organism and environment. The arterial blood gases are the net result of the schema's "checks and balances." It would be clinically advantageous to be able to predict the changes a given disease is likely to produce in this schema and also to predict the effects of supportive therapy. In other words, to apply blood gas measurements clinically we must know the physiologic effects of cardiopulmonary disease on the homeostatic schema.

The radiologist and pathologist classify cardiopulmonary disease anatomically; for example, pneumonia is classified as lobar, bronchial, or interstitial. The chest physician classifies the same disease either by etiology (bacterial, viral) or by pulmonary function (restrictive, obstructive). Each clinical discipline classifies the disease according to the measurements, clinical assessments, and therapies available to it. In the disciplines of respiratory care and critical-care medicine, blood gas measurements are used to reflect the physiologic status of the cardiopulmonary system. Therefore, the anesthesiologist, the critical-care physician, the nurse, and the respiratory therapist must classify cardiopulmonary diseases physiologically.

Cardiopulmonary pathophysiology may be divided into two major categories: *shunt-producing disease* and *deadspace-producing disease*. Physiologic deadspace may be measured by the deadspace/tidal volume ratio (see Chapter 8), and intrapulmonary shunting may be directly measured (see Chapter 19). These measurements and calculations are often not feasible in the acutely ill patient for whom immediate supportive measures are indicated. We must learn to recognize deadspace disease or shunting disease by means of blood gas analysis and clinical evaluation. Familiarity with this approach will make the clinical application of blood gas analysis meaningful and appropriate.

Table 16–1 outlines a general physiologic classification of cardiopulmonary disease. This list must not be considered complete or absolute; it is intended as a general clinical guideline. The text considers the listed abnormalities in some detail and the chapter concludes with a discussion of some general diagnostic guidelines.

Deadspace-Producing Disease

Deadspace ventilation is grossly reflected in a *minute volume-arterial carbon dioxide tension disparity* (see Chapter 12).[214] We may

TABLE 16–1.—PHYSIOLOGIC CLASSIFICATION OF
CARDIOPULMONARY DISEASE

I. Deadspace producing	II. Shunt producing
A. Anatomic	A. Anatomic
1. Rapid, shallow breathing	1. Congenital heart disease
	2. Intrapulmonary fistula
	3. Vascular lung tumor
B. Alveolar deadspace	B. Capillary shunting
1. Acute pulmonary embolus	1. Acute atelectasis
2. Decreased pulmonary per-	2. Alveolar fluid
fusion	
a. Decreased cardiac output	
b. Acute pulmonary hyper-	
tension	
C. Deadspace effect	C. Shunt effect
(ventilation in excess of per-	(perfusion in excess of ventilation;
fusion)	venous admixture)
1. Alveolar septal destruction	1. Hypoventilation
2. Positive-pressure ventilation	2. Uneven distribution of ventilation
	3. Diffusion defect

postulate that a nonexercising, spontaneously breathing person with a 6 L minute volume possesses an arterial carbon dioxide tension of 40 mm Hg. If the minute volume is increased to 12 L and cardiac output increases proportionately, the arterial P_{CO_2} will be approximately 30 mm Hg; if the minute volume is increased to 24 L, the arterial carbon dioxide tension will be in the 20 mm Hg range (see Chapter 12).

Anatomic Deadspace Disease

Anatomic deadspace is normally constant and predictable — approximately 1 ml/pound (2.2 ml/kg) of normal body weight. The major cause of increased anatomic deadspace is *rapid, shallow breathing,* which most often results from either of two pathophysiologic conditions: increased work of breathing or central nervous system malfunction.

Increased work of breathing. — Increased physiologic deadspace, decreased lung compliance, increased airway resistance, or significantly decreased vital capacity increases the work of breathing (see Chapter 11). The body's basic mechanism for conserving ventilatory energy is to breathe a smaller tidal volume, which uses a smaller percentage of vital capacity for tidal volume (see Chapter 11). The need to provide an adequate alveolar ventilation causes ventilatory frequency to increase as tidal volume decreases.[215]

Central nervous system malfunction. — A central nervous system depression (e.g., anesthesia, sedation, or poisoning) usually leads to a rapid, shallow breathing pattern. Central nervous system disease (e.g., brain tumor or increased cerebral spinal fluid pressure) may similarly affect the ventilatory pattern.

An obvious exception is narcotic overdose, which causes a very deep and slow breathing pattern.

Alveolar Deadspace Disease

The two most common clinical causes are acute pulmonary embolus and acutely decreased pulmonary perfusion.

ACUTE PULMONARY EMBOLUS. — This acutely produces ventilated but unperfused alveoli. It is the classic example of alveolar deadspace disease.[218, 219] Some have classified this as a shunting disease because it usually is *accompanied by arterial hypoxemia.*[216] The hypoxemia is due in part to concomitant venous admixture, increased work of breathing, decreased cardiac output, and other factors which are poorly understood.[217]

Acute pulmonary embolus often results in cardiopulmonary collapse. In patients who have the cardiopulmonary reserves to meet the stress, increased minute volume is the rule—an increase that is usually far greater than can be accounted for by the relatively small increase in alveolar ventilation, i.e., a significant MV-Pa_{CO_2} disparity exists (see Chapter 12). There is no such thing as "typical" blood gases in acute pulmonary embolus.

ACUTELY DECREASED PULMONARY PERFUSION. —This is most commonly due to two factors in the critically ill patient:

1. *Acutely decreased cardiac output.*—This causes a relatively greater portion of the cardiac output to flow through the gravity-dependent areas of the lung (see Chapter 7).[12] This uneven distribution of perfusion increases areas of ventilated but unperfused lung. *Clinically, this is perhaps the single most common cause of acutely increased deadspace ventilation.*[220] Whenever there is clinical evidence of acutely decreased cardiac output, one must be concerned with increased work of breathing secondary to deadspace ventilation increase. The hypoxemia that accompanies decreased cardiac output is primarily due to decreased mixed venous oxygen content (see Chapters 6 and 9).

2. *Acute pulmonary hypertension.*—Because of acutely increased pulmonary vascular resistance, the right heart cardiac output tends to be acutely decreased. Thus, acute pulmonary hypertension leads to increased deadspace ventilation.[80] Acute pulmonary hypertension is most commonly caused by acidemia, low alveolar oxygen tensions, and severe arterial hypoxemia (see Chapter 7).

Deadspace Effect — Ventilation in Excess of Perfusion

Two possible physiologic conditions may occur in alveoli that have ventilation in excess of perfusion. First, there may be increased exchange of gases, which causes an increase in alveolar ventilation (a decreased arterial carbon dioxide tension). Second, the excessive ventilation may not exchange with blood, and this causes an increase in deadspace ventilation. Obviously, the outcome of any given circumstance of ventilation in excess of perfusion is unpredictable, infinitely complex, and ever changing. There are, basically, two common clinical situations in which ventilation in excess of perfusion may be significant: alveolar septal destruction and positive-pressure ventilation.

ALVEOLAR SEPTAL DESTRUCTION. — This is most commonly found in the septal alveolar wall degeneration of emphysema where large single air sacs replace several alveoli.[1] Due to the loss of surface area for gas exchange, much of the total ventilation does not exchange with blood.

POSITIVE-PRESSURE VENTILATION. — This is most commonly encountered with the use of a volume ventilator or during general anesthesia, when significantly increasing minute ventilation is not accompanied by corresponding increases in cardiac output.[129, 221] In addition, there is a preference for the delivered gas to be distributed to the more poorly perfused lung areas.[222] Therefore, much of the increased total ventilation is deadspace because there has been no concomitant increase in pulmonary blood flow.[223]

Shunt-Producing Disease

Most physicians and allied health personnel equate hypoxemia with shunting. Although the two are related, the effect of any shunt on arterial oxygen tension is directly proportional to the degree of hemoglobin concentration and saturation of the shunted blood (see Chapter 9). Any uncompensated increase in metabolic rate or any uncompensated decrease in cardiac output will decrease the mixed venous oxygen content, thereby accentuating the degree of hypoxemia resulting from the shunt (see Chapters 9 and 19).

Anatomic Shunting Disease

Anatomic shunting is the flow of blood from the right heart to the left heart without going through the pulmonary capillaries. Three common categories of disease cause this condition:

CONGENITAL HEART DISEASE. — Any congenital heart defect that results in a right-to-left flow of blood produces an anatomic shunt.

INTRAPULMONARY FISTULAS. — These may be congenital or they may result from chest trauma or disease.

VASCULAR LUNG TUMORS. — Lung tumors can become quite vascular. When they do so, pulmonary arterial blood is able to pass through the tumor mass and into the pulmonary veins without coming into contact with alveoli.

Capillary Shunting Disease

ACUTE ATELECTASIS. — This is by far the most common clinical cause of absolute shunting. The causes of acute atelectasis include the following: (1) space-occupying lesions of the chest, e.g., pneumothorax, hemothorax, and pleural fluid — these entities press on lung tissue and cause *compression* atelectasis; (2) total obstruction of bronchi and/or bronchioles, causing absorption of the distal alveolar air — *absorption* atelectasis; and (3) microatelectasis — the random collapse of alveoli resulting from constant volume ventilation or increased surface tension (e.g., adult respiratory distress syndrome).

ALVEOLAR FLUID. — Usually it is the result of alveolar abscess, gross pulmonary edema, pneumonia, or pooled secretions.

Shunt Effect — Perfusion in Excess of Ventilation

This is also known as *venous admixture* or *ventilation/perfusion inequality*. It is the shunting phenomenon that is most readily correctable by oxygen therapy.

HYPOVENTILATION. — This is a common cause of hypoxemia. Obviously, hypoventilation results in a decreased alveolar gas delivery. At room air this means a less than normal oxygenation of the blood that is exchanging with the alveolar air.[207]

UNEVEN DISTRIBUTION OF VENTILATION. — This is a common cause of alveolar hypoventilation (see Chapter 7). The underventilated alveoli have a drop in oxygen tension, which results in suboxygenation of blood flowing past these alveoli. *This kind of venous admixture occurs in almost all pulmonary diseases.*[99] It is certainly a prime reason for hypoxemia in chronic obstructive pulmonary disease.

DIFFUSION DEFECTS. — These are diseases in which the alveolar-capillary membrane is altered so that diffusion of all gas molecules is impeded. Under certain circumstances this means that the blood passing by the alveolus does not have time to equilibrate with the alveolar oxygen tension. This causes an increase in the alveolar-arterial oxygen tension difference $(A-aD_{O_2})$, and hypoxemia ensues.[135] Essentially, the diffusion impedance creates a situation in which the gradient between the alveolar oxygen tension and the pulmonary capillary blood is not sufficient to provide equilibration in the time allotted.

Diffusion defects cannot be readily distinguished from shunt effect in the critically ill patient because diffusion tests and/or exercise tests are not practical. For the purpose of supportive cardiopulmonary care, diffusion defects may be classified as shunt effect because the hypoxemia is highly responsive to oxygen therapy; that is, increasing the alveolar oxygen tension will improve the alveolar to capillary oxygen gradient.

Diagnostic Use of Blood Gas Analysis

Arterial blood gas measurements do not rule out cardiopulmonary disease; rather, they reflect the net result of the cardiopulmonary disease minus the compensatory mechanisms of the cardiopulmonary system. In other words, *we may see near normal blood gases in the presence of significant cardiopulmonary disease, as well as abnormal blood gases that do not totally reflect the severity of the cardiopulmonary disease because of compensatory mechanisms.*

Blood gas analysis may be helpful in ruling out certain disease categories by differentiating shunt-producing disease from deadspace-producing disease. To illustrate this point, let us consider the following case studies.

A 40-year-old, 110-pound woman with thrombophlebitis of the right leg for two days suddenly complains of chest pain and shortness of breath:

FI_{O_2} 21%

pH	7.52	VT	400 ml	BP	140/70
PCO_2	27 mm Hg	RR	30/min	P	110/min
PO_2	60 mm Hg	MV	12L	T	100°F

The interpretation is "acute alveolar hyperventilation with mild hypoxemia." The more than twice normal minute volume is reflected in the greatly increased alveolar ventilation. This *tends to rule out* acute deadspace disease.*

---

*Of course, multiple small pulmonary emboli may occur over a period of days without producing clinically detectable deadspace ventilation increases.

Now consider the following data in the same patient after 20 minutes of oxygen therapy:

FI_{O_2} 50%

pH	7.48	V_T	400 ml	BP	120/80
PCO_2	33 mm Hg	RR	20/min	P	90/min
PO_2	90 mm Hg	MV	8 L	T	100°F

At 50% inspired oxygen the ventilatory and myocardial work have been decreased. This is typical of acute alveolar hyperventilation due to hypoxemia (see Chapter 15) — i.e., it is more commonly the result of a shunt-producing disease. In fact, this woman had a pneumonia in in the left lower lobe. Of course, blood gas measurements *alone* did not rule out pulmonary embolus, but they were *consistent* with that conclusion.

If the diagnosis were pulmonary embolus, the following data would have been more typical:

FI_{O_2} 21%

pH	7.48	V_T	600 ml	BP	140/70
PCO_2	33 mm Hg	RR	25/min	P	110/min
PO_2	60 mm Hg	MV	15 L	T	100°F

FI_{O_2} 50%

pH	7.45	V_T	600 ml	BP	120/70
PCO_2	35 mm Hg	RR	25/min	P	100/min
PO_2	80 mm Hg	MV	15 L	T	100°F

The minute volume is about three times normal and yet the alveolar ventilation is in the low normal range. This suggests increased deadspace ventilation. At 50% inspired oxygen, the significant increase in arterial oxygenation without significant changes in the ventilatory status is *suggestive* of deadspace-producing disease and *tends to rule out* shunt-producing disease.

These examples are clear-cut for teaching purposes. Clinically, the situation may be extremely complex and many factors may be involved. The following guidelines will prove beneficial in the vast majority of clinical circumstances; however, the reader should keep in mind that exceptions are not uncommon.

Guidelines for Acute Deadspace-Producing Diseases

1. Minute volume increases greatly with little or no response in alveolar ventilation (MV − MVA = MVD).
2. Changes in total ventilation are minimal in response to oxygen therapy, whereas increases in arterial oxygen tensions may be dramatic.

3. Accurate deadspace/tidal volume ratio measurements are technically difficult to obtain and of relatively little value in the presence of tachypnea.

Guidelines for Acute Shunt-Producing Diseases

1. Increased minute ventilation is directly reflected in alveolar ventilation.
2. When cardiopulmonary reserves are adequate to meet the stress:
   a. The blood gas measurements will usually show an acute alveolar hyperventilation with hypoxemia.
   b. Clinical evidence of increased cardiovascular work is present, e.g., hypertension and tachycardia.
3. Assuming the hypoxemia is at least partially responsive to oxygen therapy (i.e., at least some venous admixture is present), appropriate oxygen therapy results in:
   a. A decreased work of breathing as reflected in decreased ventilatory rate, decreased use of accessory muscles of ventilation, a subjective feeling of improvement, and Pa_{CO_2} increased toward normal.
   b. Decreased myocardial work as reflected in a decrease of hypertension, a decrease in tachycardia, and the disappearance or diminishment in frequency of ventricular premature beats when present.
   c. *Significantly improved arterial oxygen tensions,* but only after the work of breathing and the myocardial work have been reduced significantly.

17 / Common Clinical Causes of Abnormal Blood Gases

THE INTERPRETATIVE GUIDELINES described in Chapters 12, 13, and 14 enable us to place cardiopulmonary and acid-base pathophysiology within certain categories. These categories are most useful as guides to acute clinical support; but, in addition, they can help us to make differential diagnoses. This chapter discusses the more common clinical diseases from the standpoint of blood gas measurement. The diseases are considered in accordance with the following outline (which includes page numbers for future reference):

I. Metabolic Acid-Base Imbalance

Metabolic acid-base imbalance is common in the critically ill patient. Unfortunately, it is often missed or misjudged clinically until the condition is severe. The clinical availability of blood gas measurements has allowed direct measurement of blood pH and PCO_2. Easy access to this information has allowed the clinician to be alerted to minor changes in pH and blood base. Thus, most of the mystery and complexity that formerly surrounded clinical acid-base imbalance has been removed.

Acidosis and alkalosis are pathophysiologic processes in which the normal quantities of acid and base are skewed (see Chapter 10). When metabolic *acidemia* or *alkalemia* is present, it denotes that the metabolic process is *uncompensated.* We have delineated *acidemia* as an arterial pH below 7.30 (see Chapter 12); it may be life threatening by itself because: (1) enzyme systems do not function properly; (2) myocardial and central nervous system electrophysiology may be interfered with; (3) electrolyte balance may be acutely upset; (4) acute pulmonary hypertension may be manifested; and (5) autonomic receptors may not react predictably to exogenous drugs. *Alkalemia* has been delineated as a pH of more than 7.50 and in and of itself may be threatening to life-supporting systems (see Chapter 12).

The support and correction of metabolic acidemia and metabolic alkalemia are clinical questions separate from the therapeutics of the underlying pathophysiologic processes of metabolic acidosis and metabolic alkalosis. At this time we shall consider the common causes of metabolic acidosis and metabolic alkalosis. The reader must keep in mind that the severity of the accompanying acidemia or alkalemia must be considered as a separate clinical question.

A. Metabolic Acidosis

This is the result of the loss of blood base or the accumulation of excessive nonvolatile blood acid, or both. With the exception of lactic acidosis, metabolic acidosis is rarely due to primary pulmonary disease. It usually elicits a compensatory alveolar hyperventilation (decreased Pa_{CO_2}). Hypoxemia is rare as long as the cardiovascular status remains adequate.

TYPICAL ROOM AIR BLOOD GASES
    pH   Below 7.40
    P_{CO_2} Below 40 mm Hg
    P_{O_2} Above 80 mm Hg
    Plasma bicarbonate usually less than normal.
    Base excess always negative.
TYPICAL VENTILATORY PATTERN
    VT   Eupnea (normal depth) or hyperpnea (deeper than normal)
    RR   Tachypnea (rapid frequency)
    MV   Above normal
GENERAL RESPONSE TO OXYGEN THERAPY
    1. Dramatic increase in Pa_{O_2}.
    2. Ventilatory state relatively unchanged.
EVALUATION OF TISSUE OXYGENATION
    1. Oxygen content decreased from normal (shift to the right).
    2. Cardiovascular status is the prime determinant of tissue oxygenation.
    3. If hypoxemia is present, *hypoxia must be assumed.*

1. RENAL FAILURE (RENAL TUBULAR ACIDOSIS).—The inadequate renal function means that the normal metabolic waste products are not being excreted adequately. Depending on whether the problem is tubular or glomerular, some combination of accumulation of blood acid and decrease of blood base occurs.[224] Primarily there is a disruption of hydrogen ion excretion.

When the diagnosis of renal failure or renal tubular acidosis is made, attention must be paid to the patient's ability to compensate by increasing ventilatory work. A lack of adequate ventilatory reserve or the onset of fatigue could make the acidosis far more life threatening.

Renal acidosis is generally slow in onset and is seldom accompanied by a significant acidemia.

2. KETO-ACIDOSIS (DIABETIC ACIDOSIS OR STARVATION).—Normal cellular metabolism requires both sugar and oxygen to produce energy. Insulin is essential for the transport of glucose into the cell. When the diabetic patient has a deficit of blood insulin, the glucose cannot adequately enter the cell; therefore alternate cellular pathways of metabolism are utilized. The same process occurs when glucose is unavailable due to starvation. The metabolites of the alternate pathways are ketones and the result is a keto-acidosis (see Chapter 10).

This patient is usually quite capable of generating a great deal of ventilatory work, and therefore he achieves a state of hyperpnea (deep breaths) and tachypnea (rapid breathing)—referred to as *Kussmaul breathing*. This typical "total hyperventilation" of diabetic acidosis is an important diagnostic sign.

3. **LACTIC ACIDOSIS.**—Metabolism continues through metabolic pathways known as *anaerobic pathways* when oxygen is unavailable to tissues (see Chapter 6). The metabolic products of these pathways —lactate ion and hydrogen ion—form a nonvolatile acid (lactic acid) in the blood, which has a profound effect on the blood pH.

A severe drop in cardiac output, circulatory shutdown, or severe hypoxemia may result in the accumulation of lactic acid.[225] This is the rule in the patient with profound cardiopulmonary collapse! Lactic acidosis usually dissipates rapidly with the reestablishment of circulation, ventilation, and oxygenation (see Chapter 10).

B. Metabolic Alkalosis

Metabolic alkalosis is quite common in the critically ill patient. Although not as directly life threatening as metabolic acidosis, metabolic alkalosis has a dire potential. The immediate compensatory mechanism for metabolic alkalosis is a decrease in ventilatory work (compensatory alveolar hypoventilation); this compensation may be severe enough to cause hypoxemia. It is rare for metabolic alkalosis to cause a "significant" decrease in alveolar ventilation in an alert patient; the tendency is for the alkalemia to remain uncompensated. In the unconscious, semicomatose, or severely debilitated patient, however, metabolic alkalosis may precipitate a marked alveolar hypoventilation.[226]

TYPICAL ROOM AIR BLOOD GASES
  pH   Above 7.40
  Pco_2 Above 40 mm Hg
  Po_2 60–100 mm Hg
  Plasma bicarbonate usually above normal.
  Base excess always positive.
TYPICAL VENTILATORY PATTERN
  V_T Usually eupnea or mild hypopnea (shallow breaths)
  RR   Normal or bradypnea (slow frequency)
GENERAL RESPONSE TO OXYGEN THERAPY
  1. Dramatic increase in Pa_{O_2}.
  2. Ventilatory state relatively unchanged.
EVALUATION OF TISSUE OXYGENATION
  1. Oxygen content increased (shift to the left); hemoglobin-oxygen affinity increased.
  2. If significant hypoxemia is present, the tissue oxygenation state depends on the adequacy of the cardiovascular system.

1. **Hypokalemia.**—This condition is most commonly found after several days of intravenous therapy in which potassium replacement has been inadequate. Diuretic therapy and diarrhea are other common causes of hypokalemia.[227]

Total body potassium depletion results in metabolic alkalosis by two important mechanisms:

a. The kidneys attempt to conserve potassium, resulting in hydrogen ion excretion and a concomitant increase in blood base.

b. Potassium (K^+) is the major intracellular cation. Total body depletion induces intracellular potassium to enter the extracellular space in an attempt to maintain near normal serum levels. As potassium leaves the cell, hydrogen ion must enter. This leads to an increase in blood base.

The measurement of abnormally low potassium ion contents in the serum (hypokalemia) usually reflects a severe depletion of total body potassium. Low normal levels of serum potassium may be maintained in the presence of significant total body potassium depletion. Thus, the metabolic alkalosis (and other manifestations of potassium depletion) may be present while *serum* potassium levels are maintained in the low normal range. As a general rule, abnormally low potassium levels (hypokalemia) reflect a *severe* loss of total body potassium.

Clinically, hypokalemia is manifested as (1) metabolic alkalosis, (2) muscular weakness, and (3) cardiac arrhythmia. *This is a most significant triad in a patient with a borderline ventilatory reserve.* In addition, potassium deficit may precipitate digitalis intoxication.

2. **Hypochloremia.**—The chloride ion (Cl^-) is the major anion of the body electrolytes; when depleted, the bicarbonate ion must increase in concentration to maintain electrical balance with the cations (see Chapter 10). Thus, decreased blood chloride concentration usually leads to increased blood bicarbonate concentrations.

In addition, the chloride ion is the major exchangeable anion for the renal tubules. If adequate chloride ion is not available, tubular exchange is hindered and usually results in additional potassium loss.[228, 229]

3. **Gastric suction or vomiting.**—The primary insult is loss of hydrochloric acid (HCl), but this is soon compounded by potassium loss in the kidney and the gastrointestinal tract.

A common mistake is to attempt to reverse this metabolic alkalosis by administration of ammonium chloride. This adds to sodium and potassium loss, and the patient deteriorates. Replacement of chloride, water, and potassium will allow the kidneys to reverse the metabolic alkalosis.[228]

4. **Massive administration of steroids.** — This is not unusual therapy in critically ill patients. High dosage of sodium-retaining steroids leads to accelerated excretion of hydrogen ion and potassium in the distal tubules of the kidney, and the result is metabolic alkalosis. Newer steroid preparations, such as methylprednisolone sodium succinate (Solumedrol), have little tendency for sodium retention and therefore manifest little, if any, metabolic alkalosis problems in massive doses.

5. **Sodium bicarbonate administration.** — Metabolic alkalosis often occurs after cardiopulmonary resuscitation. Although many factors are involved, certainly one must consider excessive administration of sodium bicarbonate a major factor. However, intact kidneys have a great ability to excrete the excess bicarbonate — as long as there is no potassium depletion.

II. Alveolar Hyperventilation (Respiratory Alkalosis)

Alveolar hyperventilation may or may not be secondary to pulmonary disease. Blood gas analysis is most helpful in delineating the etiology because there are only *three physiologic causes of alveolar hyperventilation:* (1) chemoreceptor response to arterial hypoxemia (see Chapter 9), (2) ventilatory response to metabolic acidosis, and (3) central nervous system malfunction.

Alveolar hyperventilation due to hypoxemia. — This is typically a Pa_{CO_2} between 25 and 35 mm Hg, accompanied by a moderate hypoxemia; i.e., the room air Pa_{O_2} is between 40 and 80 mm Hg. To help determine if the hypoxemia is the cause of the alveolar hyperventilation, one must test the response to oxygen therapy. If the alveolar hyperventilation is secondary to hypoxemia, oxygen therapy will:

1. Decrease alveolar ventilation; i.e., arterial carbon dioxide tension will increase toward normal and the work of breathing will decrease.
2. Decrease the heart rate if tachycardia is present.
3. Decrease the blood pressure if hypertension is present.

Arterial oxygen tensions will seldom increase above 80 mm Hg with proper oxygen therapy.

Alveolar hyperventilation due to metabolic acidosis. — This is due to the homeostatic response of attempting to create a respiratory alkalemia to normalize the acid pH. The blood gas findings should immediately reveal the situation: the pH will be less than 7.40, plasma bicarbonate will be less than normal, and the base deficit will be significant. These findings are to be interpreted as *metabolic acidosis,* since that is the primary pathophysiology. The ventilatory response—alveolar hyperventilation—is secondary.

Alveolar hyperventilation due to "central causes."—This category is reached only after the first two have been ruled out. Such factors as trauma, central nervous system infection, primary brain lesions, systemic sepsis, lung stretch receptor stimulation, and central nervous system depression may lead to central nervous system stimulation of ventilation. As a general rule these patients do not have pulmonary disease, and in response to oxygen therapy they have dramatic rises in arterial P_{O_2} with little change in ventilatory status.

Immediate clinical assessment of alveolar hyperventilation must center on cardiopulmonary reserve, inasmuch as both the work of breathing and myocardial work are increased. Supportive measures such as oxygen therapy must be instituted while rapid diagnosis of the underlying disease process is being carried out. We will consider the disease entities under three main headings: (1) acute alveolar hyperventilation with hypoxemia, (2) chronic alveolar hyperventilation with hypoxemia, (3) alveolar hyperventilation without hypoxemia.

A. Acute Alveolar Hyperventilation with Hypoxemia

TYPICAL ROOM AIR BLOOD GASES
   pH   Above 7.50
   P_{CO_2} Below 35 mm Hg; below 30 mm Hg when clinically
                  significant
   P_{O_2} 40–80 mm Hg
   Plasma bicarbonate within normal range.
   Base excess within normal range.
TYPICAL VENTILATORY PATTERN
   VT   Hyperpnea (deep)
   RR   Tachypnea (rapid)
   MV   Greater than normal
   Dyspnea frequent.
GENERAL RESPONSE TO OXYGEN THERAPY
   1. Little rise in Pa_{O_2}.
   2. Decreased ventilatory work (increased Pa_{CO_2}).
   3. Decreased myocardial work.
EVALUATION OF TISSUE OXYGENATION
   Hypoxia is rare as long as ventilatory and myocardial reserves do not
   fail.

1. **ACUTE PULMONARY DISEASE.** — This category includes pneumo-

nia and atelectasis, adult respiratory distress syndrome (ARDS), and acute asthma.

a. Pneumonia and atelectasis. — When acute alveolar hyperventilation with hypoxemia is due to an acute pulmonary disease, it is most commonly due to a combination of pneumonia and atelectasis. Almost all acute pulmonary diseases lead to inflammatory changes in the tracheobronchial tree and the alveoli; and this in turn leads to collapse of alveoli, pooling of secretions, and uneven distribution of ventilation.[11] The resulting intrapulmonary shunt causes arterial hypoxemia. The ventilatory system increases its work to compensate for the hypoxemia and in so doing causes a decrease in arterial Pco_2.

The following are groups of patients who commonly manifest pneumonia and atelectasis. These, of course, are in addition to the large number of patients who present with primary pulmonary infection.

(1) Patients who have had abdominal or thoracic operations are unable to breathe as deeply or cough as effectively as they were able to do before operation; i.e., vital capacity is greatly decreased.[230] The disability is due primarily to peritoneal irritation, and it results in the pooling of normally produced secretions and the collapse of alveoli at the base of the lung. This combination of microatelectasis and pneumonia is often called *stasis pneumonia.* Acute alveolar hyperventilation with hypoxemia is common in the first several postoperative days.[231] Oxygen therapy is almost always indicated during this period, as is proper bronchial hygiene therapy.[11]

(2) Traumatized patients manifest similar pulmonary problems. If the trauma is causing pain that restricts the ability to cough and to breathe deeply, or if the trauma is to the central nervous system so that the patient has been rendered unconscious, microatelectasis and pneumonia will eventually occur. This may be avoided by *early* application of proper respiratory therapy.

(3) Patients with neurologic diseases may have muscular weakness that produces an inability to cough and deep breathe effectively. This leads to atelectasis and pneumonia if aggressive respiratory therapy is not instituted.

(4) Patients who aspirate foreign bodies into the tracheobronchial tree have significant atelectasis and, eventually, pneumonia.

(5) Segmental or lobar atelectasis is common in many debilitated patients. The sudden onset of fever, dyspnea, and hypoxemia are the usual clinical signs of an acute major atelectasis. The blood gas measurements usually show acute alveolar hyperventilation with hypoxemia.

b. Adult respiratory distress syndrome (ARDS). — This general syndrome is described under many names in the medical literature, primarily because of its numerous etiologies. Among the best-known descriptive terms are post-traumatic pulmonary insufficiency, shock lung, stiff lung, oxygen toxicity, and ventilator lung. ARDS is a physiologic triad of increasing intrapulmonary shunting, decreasing lung compliance, and increasing work of breathing.[232] The entity is marked by an insidious onset of alveolar hyperventilation and increasing hypoxemia. This is not often detected clinically until the process is quite severe; that is, when profound cardiopulmonary collapse is imminent.[233] As blood gas analysis has been more commonly used and understood in acute supportive medicine, the recognition of ARDS has been made earlier in its course and, one hopes, early supportive preventive measures instituted.

c. Acute asthma. — The asthmatic patient in the acute phase has a sudden increase in airway resistance due to bronchospasm and thick, tenacious secretions. Unevenness of distribution of ventilation creates a great deal of venous admixture, which results in a mild arterial hypoxemia.[1] The patient usually is capable of producing enough ventilatory work to provide an increased alveolar ventilation in response to the hypoxemia. *Air trapping* further increases the work of breathing.

The acute asthmatic who is retaining carbon dioxide is undergoing extreme fatigue that threatens his life; in other words, *ventilatory failure in the acute asthmatic is a dire circumstance.*[234] The acute asthmatic attack is typified by acute alveolar hyperventilation with hypoxemia.

2. ACUTE MYOCARDIAL DISEASE. — In acute myocardial disease the blood gases usually are close to normal or else show acute alveolar hyperventilation with hypoxemia. The primary cardiopulmonary manifestation of the acute myocardial insult is a decreased cardiac output. Because the metabolic rate stays the same while the capillary blood flow rate decreases, there is a drop in mixed venous oxygen content (see Chapters 6, 9, and 19); therefore any pre-existing intrapulmonary shunt has a far greater hypoxemic effect on the arterial blood. Inasmuch as the cardiovascular system is not capable of readily increasing cardiac output in response to the hypoxemia, the ventilatory system attempts to compensate by increasing the alveolar ventilation. The result is acute alveolar hyperventilation with hypoxemia.

The following is a discussion of the most common cardiopulmonary problems of primary myocardial disease causing acute alveolar hyperventilation with hypoxemia.

a. Acute myocardial infarction. — The typical blood gases of a patient with an acute myocardial infarction may be near normal or else show acute alveolar hyperventilation with mild hypoxemia. The hypoxemic patient has a tachypnea and a mild hyperpnea, along with a tachycardia and usually mild hypertension (although hypotension is not uncommon). The ventilatory system is doing much of the compensatory work in response to the hypoxemia, which is secondary to venous admixture plus decreased central venous oxygen content.

These patients benefit greatly from proper oxygen therapy, even when hypoxemia is mild.[235] The benefit is believed to be twofold: a decreased work demand on the injured myocardium and a decreased demand for ventilatory work.

b. Pulmonary edema. — This entity actually consists of two separate clinical problems.

(1) Various diseases can cause an accumulation of fluid in the alveolar-capillary space — the condition known as *interstitial pulmonary edema.*[236] The result is oxygen diffusion impedance and decreased lung compliance. This basic diffusion problem results in a mild arterial hypoxemia, to which the cardiovascular and ventilatory systems respond by increasing work. In many instances the cardiovascular system is unable to respond to any great degree; therefore most of the compensatory work is undertaken by the ventilatory system. Obviously, then, alveolar ventilation is greatly increased, and the result is acute alveolar hyperventilation with hypoxemia. The overall response to oxygen therapy is usually dramatic.

(2) In *gross pulmonary edema* a transudation of fluid into the alveolar spaces occurs.[236] The condition may therefore be considered the severe form of interstitial edema. Four basic mechanisms can contribute to this edema: *(a)* increased pulmonary capillary hydrostatic pressure secondary to left heart failure or a marked increase in pulmonary artery pressure without arteriolar constriction; *(b)* decreased oncotic pressure in the pulmonary capillary blood, secondary to hypoproteinemia and related diseases; *(c)* decreased alveolar pressures, secondary to upper airway obstruction; and *(d)* destruction of or damage to the alveolar-capillary membrane, secondary to an insult such as inhalation burn.

By far the most common cause of gross pulmonary edema is left heart failure.[236, 238] The respiratory supportive measures in any pulmonary edema are basically two: proper oxygen therapy and positive pressure ventilation.

Bubbles forming in the alveoli and the bronchi are the immediate problem in gross pulmonary edema. The foaming prevents much of the air that is moving in and out of the lungs from exchanging with the pulmonary blood. In an attempt to overcome the decreased oxygen tension in the "trapped" alveolar air, the pulmonary system attempts to increase air exchange. Thus, gross pulmonary edema usually presents as acute alveolar hyperventilation with severe hypoxemia.

In addition to specific corrective measures, there are general respiratory supportive measures that usually help the patient in gross pulmonary edema: oxygen therapy, positive-pressure, and alcohol inhalation.[11]

When the insult is beyond the compensating capability of the cardiopulmonary system, acute ventilatory failure ensues — demanding far different therapy.[237] The differentiation of alveolar hyperventilation from acute ventilatory failure in the pulmonary edema patient is by blood gas measurement; clinical examination will not always correlate.

c. *Acute heart failure.* — The basic cardiopulmonary physiologic insult in heart failure is a decreased cardiac output in the face of an unchanged metabolic demand. The central venous oxygen content is decreased, and in turn this increases the hypoxemic effect of any pre-existing shunt. Because the heart is unable to increase cardiac output in response to the hypoxemic challenge, the ventilatory system responds by increasing alveolar ventilation.

Circumstances differ somewhat, depending on whether the right or the left heart has failed:

(1) In cases of *right heart failure* the alveolar hyperventilation does *not* mean the patient is in respiratory distress or dyspneic. In fact, this is uncommon in right heart failure.

If blood gases are abnormal in right heart failure, the abnormality usually is acute alveolar hyperventilation with hypoxemia. If significant venous admixture exists, oxygen therapy may make a dramatic improvement in the arterial P_{O_2}. However, this may make little difference in the state of tissue hypoxia, because tissue hypoxia is primarily dependent on cardiac output and tissue perfusion.

(2) In addition to decreased cardiac output, *left heart failure* usually includes interstitial or gross pulmonary edema.[238] It is the pulmonary edema that causes respiratory distress and dyspnea in left heart failure.

Tissue hypoxia is far more common in left heart failure, because poor perfusion of tissues is more common.

d. *Effects of cardiopulmonary bypass.* — Extracorporeal circulation (heart-lung bypass) has many physiologic complications. Generally, the lungs react to this insult by temporarily decreasing the production of surfactant. The decreased compliance, added to the peripheral vascular effects of the bypass, commonly causes a state of alveolar hyperventilation in the early postoperative period.[239] The hyperventilation usually is accompanied by a moderate hypoxemia and a mild acidemia. This combination of gas exchange abnormalities, plus the increased work of breathing caused by decreased compliance and hypoxemia, has led many physicians to believe mechanical support of ventilation is beneficial in the first 24 hours following extracorporeal circulation.

It must be remembered that alveolar hyperventilation and hypoxemia are the rule, not the exception, following heart-lung bypass.[240] Because alkalemic pH is not the rule, this entity is not actually an acute alveolar hyperventilation; however, the alveolar hyperventilation and the hypoxemia place it here more appropriately than elsewhere.

B. Chronic Alveolar Hyperventilation with Hypoxemia

TYPICAL ROOM AIR BLOOD GASES
　　pH　　　　　7.40 – 7.50
　　P_{CO_2}　　　　Below 30 mm Hg
　　P_{O_2}　　　　Below 70 mm Hg
　　Plasma bicarbonate below normal range
　　Base excess below normal range
TYPICAL VENTILATORY PATTERN
　　V_T　　　　Shallow (hypopnea)
　　RR　　　　Tachypnea
GENERAL RESPONSE TO OXYGEN THERAPY
　　1. Ventilatory status may change dramatically.
　　2. Cardiovascular status may change dramatically.
　　3. Little change in Pa_{O_2}.
EVALUATION OF TISSUE OXYGENATION
　　Hypoxia is rare as long as perfusion status remains adequate.

Chronic alveolar hyperventilation with hypoxemia is usually due to a primary pulmonary disease that is long-standing. The cardiovascular and hepatorenal systems are usually adequate in their reserves to compensate for the pulmonary state.

1. **POSTOPERATIVE CONDITIONS.** — It is common to find patients in chronic alveolar hyperventilation with hypoxemia after the second postoperative day. Any degree of pulmonary atelectasis and pneumonia causes an alveolar hyperventilation, for which the renal system will compensate in several days. Such postoperative patients usually require proper oxygen therapy in spite of their apparently excellent

clinical cardiopulmonary status. Routine evaluation for respiratory therapy is indicated.[11]

2. CHRONIC HEART FAILURE. — This is essentially the same as acute heart failure, except that the renal system has compensated and the alveolar hyperventilation with hypoxemia is now in the presence of a normal or near-normal pH. These patients have little ability to meet physiologic stress, because both the cardiac reserve and the ventilatory reserve are severely limited.

3. ADULT CYSTIC FIBROSIS. — This disease is an interesting physiologic study: a severe chronic obstructive pulmonary disease in combination with a very resilient cardiovascular system. Experience with these patients is limited, but they appear to follow a course of chronic alveolar hyperventilation with hypoxemia.[241] The advent of carbon dioxide retention is believed to be primarily due to failure of the myocardial reserve. This occurs when the pulmonary disease is so severe that total cardiopulmonary collapse is at hand. Thus, in these patients carbon dioxide retention is a dire circumstance, and death usually occurs within one year of onset.

4. THIRD-TRIMESTER PREGNANCY. — The normal respiratory physiology in the third trimester of pregnancy is a restrictive disease;[242] the vital capacity and the total lung capacity have been diminished. With the decrease in residual volume and the functional residual capacity there is a decrease in physiologic deadspace, and this causes arterial carbon dioxide tensions to fall below normal.[243] (It is also the reason these patients undergo induction of general anesthesia so rapidly.) Various endocrine changes have been postulated to play a role in the decreased arterial carbon dioxide tension.

The mild hypoxemic state is secondary to basilar atelectasis and hypoventilation, which result from the restriction of diaphragm movement by the large abdominal mass. The normal blood gas baseline in late pregnancy is chronic alveolar hyperventilation with mild hypoxemia.

5. NONCARDIOPULMONARY DISEASE. — A number of diseases can prevent normal lungs from functioning properly. Such diseases result in hypoventilation of certain portions of the lung. This hypoventilation creates venous admixture. The resulting hypoxemia is compensated both by increased cardiac output and by increased alveolar ventilation. Such patients usually manifest chronic alveolar hyperventilation with hypoxemia, and all have a decreased ventilatory reserve. We may categorize the diseases as follows:

a. Diseases causing limitation of ventilatory muscular mechanics:

(1) Neuromuscular disease, e.g., poliomyelitis, peripheral neuritis, myasthenia gravis, porphyria.

(2) Skeletal muscle disease, e.g., muscular dystrophy, myotonia.

b. Disease limiting thoracic expansion, e.g., kyphoscoliosis. Body casts and rib fracture may also have this effect.

c. Disease limiting descent of the diaphragm, e.g., peritonitis, abdominal tumor, ascites.

C. Alveolar Hyperventilation Without Hypoxemia

Alveolar hyperventilation without hypoxemia is rarely due to primary pulmonary or cardiac disease. In other words, the alveolar hyperventilation is in response to some physiologic stimulus other than hypoxemia. The stimulus may be central nervous system stimulation or insufficient oxygen *supply* to peripheral chemoreceptors; i.e., decreased oxygen-carrying capacity.

TYPICAL ROOM AIR BLOOD GASES
  pH   Above 7.40
  PCO_2 Below 30 mm Hg
  PO_2 Above minimal normal
TYPICAL VENTILATORY PATTERN
  VT   Eupnea or hyperpnea
  RR   Tachypnea
GENERAL RESPONSE TO OXYGEN THERAPY
  1. Dramatic increase in Pa_{O_2}.
  2. No significant cardiovascular or ventilatory change.
EVALUATION OF TISSUE OXYGENATION
  1. Hypoxia may be present.
  2. Oxygen transport *must* be evaluated.

1. **ANXIETY, NEUROSIS, PSYCHOSIS.** — A common cause of alveolar hyperventilation without hypoxemia is *acute anxiety*, which may be aroused by the drawing of the arterial blood, by a fear of doctors or of hospitals, and so on. This is always an *acute* alveolar hyperventilation.

True emotional disease may cause hyperventilation — this is more commonly *chronic* alveolar hyperventilation. These patients tend to be on numerous drugs, which often interreact and cause hyperventilation. Cardiopulmonary disease is rare in this kind of patient; therefore the alveolar hyperventilation is usually without hypoxemia.

2. **PAIN.** — If it does not directly restrict ventilation, pain commonly produces severe anxiety, with resultant hyperventilation. There is

good evidence to support the belief that afferent pain impulses direct-ly stimulate the respiratory centers.[3] This usually is *acute* alveolar hyperventilation without hypoxemia.

3. **CENTRAL NERVOUS SYSTEM DISEASE.** — Most intracranial disease stimulates ventilation (provided it does not produce coma). The lungs are usually nondiseased and therefore hypoxemia is rare.

4. **ANEMIA.** — In addition to acidemia, the peripheral chemorecep-tors are usually stimulated by factors that cause a reduction of the *oxy-gen supply* (see Chapter 9), such as:

a. Decreased arterial Po_2.

b. Decreased oxygen content.

c. Decreased blood flow.

A significantly decreased hemoglobin content places the major bur-den of tissue oxygenation on cardiac output; i.e., more blood must be circulated per unit of time. The chemoreceptors are more sensitive to lack of oxygen supply than are other tissues, and therefore they will be stimulated prior to other tissues experiencing hypoxia. There is rea-son to believe that chemoreceptor stimulation plays a major role in stimulating the myocardium to increase cardiac output when arterial oxygen content is low.[3]

5. **CARBON MONOXIDE POISONING.** — The carbon monoxide mole-cule has a great affinity for hemoglobin; it preferentially ties up hemo-globin sites and so prevents oxygen from attaching. Thus, carbon monoxide decreases the amount of hemoglobin available for carrying oxygen and, in so doing, decreases the oxygen content. In addition, carbon monoxide in the blood causes the hemoglobin dissociation curve to shift to the left (see Chapters 3 and 9), and thus makes the available hemoglobin far less willing to give up oxygen to the tis-sues.[5, 10, 244]

III. Deadspace Diseases

The deadspace diseases must be discussed separately, because they produce blood gas values that are meaningless if they are not com-pared with the ventilatory work (see Chapter 16).

A. Acute Pulmonary Embolus

This is the classic deadspace-producing disease — the ventilated, unperfused lung. It may be extremely difficult to diagnose clinically.

Blood gas measurements are never diagnostic, although they may help rule out acute embolic phenomena or shunt-producing disease (see Chapter 16).

Acute pulmonary embolus usually is accompanied by hypoxemia and a pH in the 7.30–7.40 range. However, blood gases may be well within acceptable ranges.

There is often a large minute volume-alveolar ventilation disparity (see Chapter 12). Several hours after the embolus, there may no longer be deadspace disease because the unperfused lung often collapses. In fact, the stasis may create collapse of perfused alveoli around the embolic area and true shunting then exists. There are no "typical" blood gases that are reflective of the pulmonary embolic phenomenon!

B. Shock (Systemic Hypotension)

Changes in the distribution of pulmonary blood flow create relatively ventilated, unperfused lung (see Chapter 7). A minute volume-alveolar ventilation disparity usually exists. The hypoxemia is primarily due to decreased central venous oxygen content, which accentuates the shunt effect.

IV. Ventilatory Failure (Respiratory Acidosis)

Ventilatory failure is defined as inadequate alveolar ventilation. This means that the patient is unable to provide enough muscular mechanical work to move a sufficient amount of air into and out of the lungs to meet the carbon dioxide metabolic demands of the body. Ventilatory failure is a severe physiologic state that must be evaluated with great care by the physician and approached with great respect by the respiratory care practitioner.

A. Chronic Ventilatory Failure (Chronic Hypercarbia)

TYPICAL ROOM AIR BLOOD GASES
    pH   7.40–7.50
    P_{CO_2} Above 50 mm Hg
    P_{O_2} Below 60 mm Hg
    Plasma bicarbonate above normal range.
    Base excess above normal range.
TYPICAL VENTILATORY PATTERN
    V_T Hypopnea (shallow)
    RR   Tachypnea (rapid)

General response to oxygen therapy
  1. *Decreased alveolar ventilation* (see Chapter 15).
  2. Sensitive to very small increases in inspired oxygen concentrations.
  3. Slight improvement in Pa_{O_2}.
Evaluation of tissue oxygenation
  1. Hypoxia is rare.
  2. Adequacy of cardiac output is the prime determinant of tissue oxygenation.
  3. Polycythemia is common; increases oxygen content.
  4. Hypoxia must be assumed if the patient becomes acidemic.

In clinical medicine the chronic hypercarbic patient is almost always the severe chronic obstructive pulmonary disease patient, i.e., emphysema and/or chronic bronchitis. Cardiopulmonary reserve is minimal and stress is life threatening.

This patient presents a particular problem to the clinician who is interpreting blood gases, because the patient is at a different baseline. Alveolar hypoventilation and hypoxemia are "baseline" values—and one judges the severity of acute disease on how the blood gases change from the baseline values. In supporting this patient, one cannot demand that he do better than he was doing prior to the acute problem; for example, if his baseline Pa_{O_2} is 50 mm Hg, one cannot try to support him at a Pa_{O_2} of 80 mm Hg, and if his baseline Pa_{CO_2} is 70 mm Hg, one cannot try to support him at a Pa_{CO_2} of 40 mm Hg (see Chapters 11 and 15).

B. Acute Alveolar Hyperventilation Superimposed on Chronic Ventilatory Failure

Typical room air blood gases
  pH   Above 7.50
  P_{CO_2} Usually above 40 mm Hg
  P_{O_2} Below 60 mm Hg
  Plasma bicarbonate usually above normal range.
  Base excess usually above normal range.
General response to oxygen therapy
  1. Proper concentrations decrease ventilatory work.
  2. Too much oxygen causes acute ventilatory failure to be superimposed on the chronic state.

The chronic hypercarbic patient may respond to acute stress by increasing alveolar ventilation. This is difficult to recognize in blood gases unless the age and clinical state of the patient are noted. The initial interpretation should be *uncompensated metabolic alkalosis with hypoxemia!* The condition must be recognized as being acute alveolar hyperventilation superimposed on a chronic ventilatory failure.

C. Acute Ventilatory Failure Superimposed on Chronic Ventilatory Failure

TYPICAL ROOM AIR BLOOD GASES
    pH   Below 7.30
    P_{CO_2} Above 60 mm Hg
    P_{O_2} Below 50 mm Hg
    Plasma bicarbonate normal or below normal.
    Base excess normal or below normal.
GENERAL RESPONSE TO OXYGEN THERAPY
    1. Proper concentration may *improve* ventilatory status.
    2. Little effect on Pa_{O_2}.
EVALUATION OF TISSUE OXYGENATION
    Hypoxia must be assumed!

It is essential to judge the severity of acute ventilatory failure on the degree of acidemia. These patients have high arterial carbon dioxide tensions with mild degrees of acidemia. This must lead to the conclusion that the patient's "baseline" state is one of high arterial P_{CO_2}.

Oxygen therapy is critical in these patients, because the proper concentrations may improve the ventilatory status and so avoid the need for a ventilator (see Chapter 15).

Oxygen therapy may have little effect on the P_{O_2} but may have a profound effect on tissue oxygenation. These patients are acute medical emergencies; tissue hypoxia must be assumed.

D. Acute Ventilatory Failure

TYPICAL ROOM AIR BLOOD GASES
    pH   Below 7.30
    P_{CO_2} Above 50 mm Hg
    P_{O_2} Below 60 mm Hg
    Plasma bicarbonate normal.
    Base excess normal.

There is no "typical ventilatory pattern." The patient may be apneic or have severe total hyperventilation.

GENERAL RESPONSE TO OXYGEN THERAPY
    1. Insignificant to mild increase in Pa_{O_2}.
    2. No change in ventilatory status.
EVALUATION OF TISSUE OXYGENATION
    Hypoxemia plus acidemia: *hypoxia must be assumed!*

This is a medical emergency! The sudden inability of a patient to move an adequate amount of air into and out of the lungs to meet carbon dioxide demands is a dire condition. This must always be considered an immediate life-threatening situation, because both hypoxemia and acidemia are present. If aggressive supportive and therapeutic measures are not undertaken, the most likely outcome is death.

18 / Support of Ventilation

TODAY'S INTENSIVE CARE SUPPORTIVE CAPABILITY includes equipment and technology that make mechanical support of ventilation feasible. No longer is placing the patient on a mechanical ventilator a "last-ditch," traumatic effort; rather, ventilator care is a sophisticated and well-defined discipline in critical-care medicine. Above all other factors, the clinical availability of arterial blood gas analysis has made modern ventilator care possible. Serial blood gas measurements are essential in the supportive care of a ventilator patient; they alone can tell us whether or not the mechanical support of ventilation is being properly applied.

The nomenclature and concepts presented in this book are based on the patient's ability to do his own work of breathing. The concept of ventilatory failure is *not applicable* when a patient is on a ventilator — the machine is providing all or part of the work of breathing. When the patient is on mechanical support of ventilation, the following terms are commonly used to evaluate the ventilatory status:

Alveolar hyperventilation	$P_{CO_2} < 30$ mm Hg
Acceptable alveolar ventilation	P_{CO_2} 30–50 mm Hg
Alveolar hypoventilation	$P_{CO_2} > 50$ mm Hg

Evaluation of the metabolic acid-base and oxygenation states on the ventilator is essentially the same as for the spontaneously breathing patient.

Ventilator Commitment

Whenever ventilator care is contemplated, it must be remembered that the underlying disease process initiating the physiologic insult must be reversible. Ventilator care is a supportive measure only! No disease is "cured" by a ventilator. Essentially, ventilator care maintains adequate cardiopulmonary homeostasis while the disease process is being arrested and reversed either by the patient's own reparative mechanisms or by appropriate medical therapeutics.

From a cardiopulmonary homeostatic viewpoint, mechanical support of ventilation may be indicated in any one of four instances:
1. *Apnea.*
2. *Acute ventilatory failure.* — Inadequate alveolar ventilation re-

213

flects an inability of the patient to move enough air into and out of the lungs to meet the carbon dioxide metabolic demands of the body. When this is accompanied by acidemia, mechanical support of ventilation is necessary, unless some other effective treatment is immediately available. The inadequate alveolar ventilation may be due to an increased deadspace ventilation (see Chapter 8), and therefore the patient may be ventilating great amounts of air (high-output failure). This may lead one to believe, falsely, that spontaneous ventilation is adequate. *The assessment of the adequacy of physiologic ventilation can be made only by blood gas analysis.*

3. *Impending acute ventilatory failure.* — This is primarily a clinical diagnosis, arrived at by assessing the work of breathing, the pathogenesis of the disease, and the patient's expected capability to *maintain* adequate ventilation. The diagnosis is often fortified by serial measurements of blood gases showing a deteriorating pattern. This assessment may be obvious, as in the patient with severe crushed chest or in the drug-overdosed patient who is rapidly becoming depressed. However, in many instances the clinical evaluation is much more difficult, e.g., in status asthmaticus or the postsurgical patient.

4. *Oxygenation.* — This is the least common of the pathophysiologic states requiring mechanical support of ventilation because most oxygenation problems are adequately supported by oxygen therapy or PEEP therapy.[11] Sometimes the support of tissue oxygenation by instituting mechanical ventilation is unsuccessful since the problem is related primarily to nonpulmonary factors. On the other hand, when hypoxemia is secondary to an acute decrease in compliance and a resultant decrease in functional residual capacity (ARDS), mechanical support of ventilation with PEEP will usually significantly improve oxygenation.[11]

Thus, arterial blood gas analysis provides invaluable information to aid in deciding whether or not ventilator support is indicated.

Ventilator Maintenance

The golden rule of mechanical ventilation is: *Obtain the best alveolar ventilation for the least cardiovascular embarrassment.* This is accomplished best when proper care is provided in three major areas:

1. *Cardiovascular stabilization.* — Alveolar ventilation is dependent upon alveolar air exchanging with pulmonary blood; therefore optimal pulmonary blood flow is as essential to proper ventilation as is any other single factor. In addition to proper fluid administration, great care must be taken to correct electrolyte imbalance and provide

myocardial support when necessary by means of such drugs as digitalis, isuprel, and dopamine. Of course, serum proteins and hemoglobin levels must be closely monitored.

2. *Acid-base balance.* — Metabolism, perfusion, and ventilation affect pH. Oxygen delivery and utilization depend greatly on pH. Meticulous care must be taken to establish and maintain acceptable hydrogen ion concentration.

3. *Ventilatory pattern.* — Cardiovascular embarrassment is directly related to intrathoracic pressures, which are indirectly related to mean airway pressures. The longer the expiratory time, the lower the mean intrathoracic pressure. Generally, *slow rates and large tidal volumes best accomplish this end.*[11]

Eucapneic Ventilation

Eucapneic ventilation means maintaining an arterial P_{CO_2} within a "normal" range — defined classically as a P_{CO_2} of between 35 and 45 mm Hg. The concept of normal ventilation should incorporate the principle of supporting the ventilatory state in the range normally maintained by the patient. A patient who normally carries an arterial P_{CO_2} of 70 mm Hg should be ventilated at an arterial P_{CO_2} of 70 mm Hg. The reasons for maintaining normal ventilation are primarily acid-base and electrolyte considerations. If an individual is maintained at an arterial P_{CO_2} significantly different from his normal range, an acute respiratory alkalosis or acidosis will result; the kidneys will respond by holding onto or getting rid of base (HCO_3^-). Normal kidneys will metabolically compensate for a ventilatory pH change in 24 to 36 hours.[13]

For example, an individual who normally carries an arterial P_{CO_2} of 70 mm Hg and a pH of 7.40 is in a state of compensated respiratory acidosis (chronic ventilatory failure); there is an excessive amount of base (HCO_3^-) present for that pH value. If this individual is suddenly ventilated and maintained at a P_{CO_2} of 40 mm Hg for several days, the kidneys will excrete this excess base to correct the sudden "respiratory alkalosis." This process causes two major problems: (1) The cardiovascular, hepatorenal, and central nervous systems will be challenged to function adequately in an alkalemic milieu and its associated electrolyte environment. Not only is cellular membrane function compromised, but sensitivities and reactivities to various drugs are less predictable and stable. The goal must be acid-base *stability* from the moment the patient is placed on the ventilator. (2) When the patient can be removed from the ventilator to assume spontaneous ventilation, he will be forced to breathe at an alveolar ventilation far greater than his pre-existent baseline state. If he assumes his previous baseline arterial PCO_2 of 70 mm Hg, he will become acidemic because the previously accumulated base excess is gone. The acute acidemia will severely challenge his limited cardiopulmonary reserves and because of his inability to maintain a state of eucapnia, the patient will end up in severe respiratory and cardiovascular distress. This often results in the patient being placed back on the ventilator and considered a "weaning problem." Note the "problem" is strictly a result of improper ventilator maintenence.

Severe acute alveolar hyperventilation can result in a decreased blood flow to the brain.[9, 10] This may be disastrous in the critically ill patient. There has been speculation that central nervous system embarrassment may be the key to major complications in ventilator care.[11]

Ventilator Discontinuance

Mechanical support of ventilation is no longer necessary when the acute disease process is sufficiently reversed and the cardiopulmonary reserves are adequate. Often essential to the evaluation of the cardiopulmonary reserves is the measurement of shunt and deadspace.[11]

Deadspace to Tidal Volume Ratio (VD/VT) Measurement

The concept of deadspace to tidal volume ratio has been discussed in chapter 8. For the patient on a volume ventilator, this measurement is reliable and easy to obtain. Its reliability makes it a useful parameter in maintaining and weaning a patient from the ventilator. With positive-pressure ventilation, the deadspace ventilation is increased because pulmonary perfusion changes in favor of gravity-dependent flow[129] and the absence of active diaphragmatic contraction favors the distribution of air to the non-gravity-dependent areas of the lung.[222] These factors are the reason why a VD/VT of less than 40% is rare in a patient on positive-pressure ventilation, and one considers a range of deadspace to tidal volume ratios between 40 and 60% as acceptable. In other words, a patient on the positive-pressure ventilator with a VD/VT of less than 60% is very likely to have a normal VD/VT ratio when spontaneously breathing.

In the absence of chronic obstructive pulmonary disease, a VD/VT ratio of greater than 80% on a volume ventilator represents a significant increase in deadspace ventilation.[2] It would mean that that patient would have to significantly increase his spontaneous ventilation above normal in order to overcome the increased deadspace. This may necessitate excessive physiologic demands due to the increased work of breathing. V_D/V_T measurements between 60% and 80% on the positive-pressure ventilator are significant and must be evaluated in relation to the other system reserves and the general clinical status of the patient.[11]

Collection of Sample for V_D/V_T

This must be a collection of *total* expired air, and it must be representative of the ventilatory pattern and its variability. In the spontaneously breathing patient this means collecting expired gas through a one-way valve system into a large collecting balloon for 5 to 10 minutes.

Experience has shown that a 5-L sample of expired gas, taken from the expiratory port of a volume ventilator, gives the same $P\bar{E}_{CO_2}$ as a 5-minute collection in a large balloon. This is undoubtedly due to the regularity of the ventilatory pattern with controlled volume ventilation.

At Northwestern Memorial Hospital we use a 5-L anesthesia bag to collect our volume ventilator samples. The bag is attached to the expiratory port as the blood gas sample is being obtained. No special apparatus or valves are needed. Caution must be taken to make sure a deep "sigh" breath is not included in the sample. When the bag is filled, it is clamped and immediately taken to the blood gas laboratory. The gas sample is then introduced into the electrode chamber and $P\bar{E}_{CO_2}$ is measured.

The Shunt Measurement

Until recently, the shunt measurement was accomplished on ventilator patients by increasing the $F_{I_{O_2}}$ to 100% for a period of 15 minutes. Recent evidence related to the effects of denitrogenation in the alveolar gas space suggests that it is more clinically meaningful to do routine measurements at an $F_{I_{O_2}}$ of 50–60%.[245, 246] In either case the following guidelines for shunt measurements on ventilator patients have proven useful over several decades:

1. A calculated shunt greater than 30% is generally considered incompatible with prolonged spontaneous ventilation.

2. Calculated shunts between 20 and 30% are considered compatible with spontaneous ventilation as long as the cardiovascular reserves are adequate and the statuses of the central nervous system and hepatorenal system are acceptable.

3. Calculated shunts less than 20% are considered completely compatible with prolonged spontaneous ventilation.

Collection of Sample for $\dot{Q}s/\dot{Q}T$

The patient is placed supine and is suctioned so that the ventilation will not be interrupted for 15 minutes. During this period the patient must not be disturbed and must be "in phase" with the ventilator. FI_{O_2} of 50% is started and is checked by oxygen analyzer.

After 15 minutes the FI_{O_2} is again checked by oxygen analyzer and vital signs are noted. Simultaneously, blood is drawn from both the arterial line and the pulmonary artery or the central venous catheter (see Chapter 20). The samples are immediately placed on ice and taken to the blood gas laboratory, where they are processed within 2 minutes. The blood gas machines are calibrated prior to the delivery of the sample.

Summary

Serial blood gas measurements are the very cornerstone of modern ventilatory support. They reflect the cardiopulmonary homeostatic status and are invaluable monitors of physiologic ventilation. In concert with pulmonary artery blood gas monitoring (see Chapter 20), the arterial measurements provide the clinician with the essential information with which to apply the technology of modern critical-care medicine.

19 / Development of the Physiologic Shunt Equation

THE PHYSIOLOGIC SHUNT is a useful concept and its measurement is often clinically helpful. Since most cardiopulmonary disease has an element of shunting, comprehension of the physiologic shunt is a practical and clinically useful tool. This chapter is devoted to a complete development of the shunt equation starting from the very basic physiology and concluding with the classic shunt equation and several modified forms used clinically. Figure 19-1 illustrates the concepts developed in this chapter.

The Fick Equation

In 1870, Adolph Fick introduced the principle of dilution methods for measuring cardiac output, with the initial example involving oxygen transport by the blood.[247] This concept has become known as the Fick principle and its initial application as the Fick equation.

A simplified development of the Fick equation is based upon the physiologic factors discussed in Chapters 6 and 9. The total quantity of oxygen potentially available for tissue consumption per unit time must include the arterial oxygen content (Ca_{O_2}) multiplied by the quantity of arterial blood presented to the tissues per unit time ($\dot{Q}T$):

$$\text{Oxygen availability} = [\dot{Q}T][Ca_{O_2}] \qquad (1)$$

The quantity of oxygen returned to the lungs is expressed as the total cardiac output ($\dot{Q}T$) multiplied by the mixed venous oxygen content ($C\bar{v}_{O_2}$):

$$\text{Oxygen returned} = [\dot{Q}T][C\bar{v}_{O_2}] \qquad (2)$$

Oxygen consumption per unit time ($\dot{V}_{O_2}$) must equal the oxygen that has been extracted from the blood in that time period; i.e., the difference between the oxygen available [equation (1)] and the oxygen returned [equation (2)]:

$$\dot{V}_{O_2} = [\dot{Q}T][Ca_{O_2}] - [\dot{Q}T][C\bar{v}_{O_2}] \qquad (3)$$

Equation (3) may be rewritten as:

$$\dot{V}_{O_2} = [\dot{Q}T][Ca_{O_2} - C\bar{v}_{O_2}] \qquad (4)$$

219

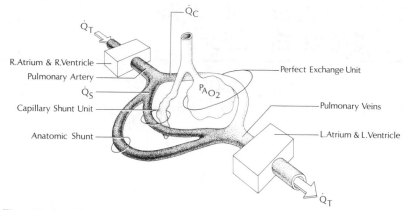

Fig 19–1.—Mathematical concept of physiologic shunting (see text). $\dot{Q}_T$ is cardiac output per unit time; $\dot{Q}_C$ is the portion of the cardiac output that exchanges perfectly with alveolar air; $\dot{Q}_S$ is the portion of the cardiac output that does not exchange with alveolar air; $P_{A_{O_2}}$ is the alveolar oxygen tension.

Equation (4) is a way of writing the Fick equation; however, it is more commonly written as:

$$\dot{Q}_T = \frac{\dot{V}_{O_2}}{[Ca_{O_2} - C\bar{v}_{O_2}]} \tag{5}$$

$\dot{Q}_T$ is cardiac output per unit time (L/min); $\dot{V}_{O_2}$ is oxygen consumption per unit time (cc/min); and $[Ca_{O_2} - C\bar{v}_{O_2}]$ is the oxygen content difference between the arterial and mixed venous blood (vol%).

Cardiac Output

The total cardiac output ($\dot{Q}_T$) is arbitrarily divided into two major components:

$$\dot{Q}_T = \dot{Q}_C + \dot{Q}_S \tag{6}$$

$\dot{Q}_C$ is the portion of the cardiac output that exchanges perfectly with alveolar air. $\dot{Q}_S$ is the portion of the cardiac output that does not exchange at all with alveolar air.

$\dot{Q}_S$ may be considered equivalent to absolute shunting (anatomic plus capillary—see Chapter 9). Where shunt effect (venous admixture) exists, the blood will be incompletely oxygenated. Therefore, that portion is divided into two components: $\dot{Q}_C$ and $\dot{Q}_S$. In other words, shunt effect is mathematically divided as though a portion of that blood exchanged perfectly and the remainder did not exchange at all.

$\dot{Q}c$ mathematically represents all the blood to which oxygen is being added as it traverses through the lung. The blood leaving these perfectly exchanging alveolar-capillary units may theoretically be said to contain an end pulmonary capillary oxygen content (Cc_{O_2}). This value is based on the assumption that complete equilibration between an alveolar gas tension and an end pulmonary capillary gas tension can exist. In those alveolar-capillary units with capillary transit times within normal ranges (0.3–0.7 sec) and alveolar oxygen tensions (PA_{O_2}) greater than 100 mm Hg, the assumption is clinically valid.[248] The "calculated" alveolar oxygen tension does not represent any real tension in the various alveoli, but represents an average value that is dependent upon the physical laws of gas exchange and the respiratory exchange ratio.

The mixed venous oxygen content represents the average blood oxygen content being returned to the lungs, and its value can be measured only in pulmonary artery blood.[9] The oxygen content of shunted blood ($\dot{Q}s$) is unchanged from the mixed venous oxygen content. The exchanging portion of the cardiac output ($\dot{Q}c$) therefore represents the only blood to which oxygen is added. It has an oxygen content referred to as end pulmonary capillary oxygen content. Therefore, the organism's oxygen consumption may also be derived from an expression written as equation (7) instead of as equation (4). Since equations (4) and (7) both equal the oxygen consumption value ($\dot{V}O_2$), they are obviously equal to each other. Therefore,

$$\dot{V}O_2 = \dot{Q}c[Cc_{O_2} - C\bar{v}_{O_2}] \tag{7}$$

$$\dot{Q}T[Ca_{O_2} - C\bar{v}_{O_2}] = \dot{Q}c[Cc_{O_2} - C\bar{v}_{O_2}] \tag{8}$$

The Classic Shunt Equation

The physiologic shunt equation expresses the relationship between the total cardiac output and the shunted cardiac output. Therefore, equation (6) is solved in terms of $\dot{Q}c$:

$$\dot{Q}c = [\dot{Q}T - \dot{Q}s] \tag{9}$$

Substituting equation (9) for $\dot{Q}c$ in equation (8) results in the following equation:

$$\dot{Q}T[Ca_{O_2} - C\bar{v}_{O_2}] = [\dot{Q}T - \dot{Q}s][Cc_{O_2} - C\bar{v}_{O_2}] \tag{10}$$

Expanding equation (10) algebraically:

$$\dot{Q}TCa_{O_2} - \dot{Q}TC\bar{v}_{O_2} = \dot{Q}TCc_{O_2} - \dot{Q}TC\bar{v}_{O_2} - \dot{Q}sCc_{O_2} + \dot{Q}sC\bar{v}_{O_2} \tag{11}$$

Note that two of the six terms $(-\dot{Q}TC\bar{v}_{O_2})$ are identical and common to both sides of the equation and therefore removed from the equation.

The collection and factoring of all $\dot{Q}s$ terms on the left side and all $\dot{Q}T$ terms on the right side of the equation result in:

$$\dot{Q}s[Cc_{O_2} - C\bar{v}_{O_2}] = \dot{Q}T[Cc_{O_2} - Ca_{O_2}] \qquad (12)$$

This relationship can now be written as a ratio of shunted cardiac output to total cardiac output:

$$\frac{\dot{Q}s}{\dot{Q}T} = \frac{[Cc_{O_2} - Ca_{O_2}]}{[Cc_{O_2} - C\bar{v}_{O_2}]} \qquad (13)$$

Equation (13) is the *classic shunt equation.*[64] It has the advantage of being derived as a ratio so that no absolute measure of cardiac output is required. In this form, the equation very clearly demonstrates that as the shunted cardiac output ($\dot{Q}s$) approaches zero, the arterial oxygen content must approach the theoretical end pulmonary capillary oxygen content. As long as a portion of the cardiac output exists as shunted blood, the arterial oxygen content will always be less than the theoretical end pulmonary capillary oxygen content. In other words, since shunted blood has the same oxygen content as mixed venous blood ($C\bar{v}_{O_2}$), when this blood mixes with the perfectly exchanging cardiac output ($\dot{Q}c$), a lowered oxygen content equilibrium must be established. This may be conceptualized as oxygen leaving the $\dot{Q}c$ hemoglobin and attaching to previously desaturated $\dot{Q}s$ hemoglobin. The end result is always an arterial oxygen content somewhere between the end pulmonary capillary oxygen content and the mixed venous oxygen content.

The Clinical Shunt Equation

The classic shunt equation [equation (13)] may be mathematically manipulated by adding and subtracting an arterial oxygen content to the denominator of the term on the right. The new form of the equation can then be written:

$$\frac{\dot{Q}s}{\dot{Q}T} = \frac{[Cc_{O_2} - Ca_{O_2}]}{[Ca_{O_2} - C\bar{v}_{O_2}] + [Cc_{O_2} - Ca_{O_2}]} \qquad (14)$$

This represents the most useful form of the clinical shunt equation because it expresses in a clearer manner the concepts and measurements applied to the clinical setting. The appearance of an arterial-mixed venous content difference in the denominator makes it quite apparent that cardiac output plays an important role in altering the result of shunted cardiac output (namely, arterial hypoxemia). It is worthwhile to expand on this point by giving an example from the clinical setting.

Arterial-Mixed Venous Oxygen Content Difference

The arterial-mixed venous oxygen content difference is directly related to the oxygen consumption and total cardiac output through the Fick equation [equation (5)]. In a critically ill patient at bedrest and supported on a ventilator, the moment-to-moment oxygen consumption may be reasonably hypothesized to remain relatively constant. In this event, changes in cardiac output may be directly related to changes in arterial-mixed venous oxygen content difference. Simply put, *as the cardiac output increases, the arterial-mixed venous oxygen content difference decreases.* As the arterial-mixed venous oxygen content difference decreases, there is usually a resultant increase in venous oxygen content. This ultimately allows for higher arterial oxygen tensions and contents because of the effect of the increased oxygen content of the shunted blood.[249] Obviously, the converse is true. The direct clinical application of this relationship may be stated as follows: The degree of arterial hypoxemia secondary to intrapulmonary shunting is reflected not only by the amount of intrapulmonary shunting that exists, but also by the organism's myocardial capability of compensating for that intrapulmonary shunting. Stated still another way, a patient with excellent myocardial reserves may frequently mask the hypoxemia of intrapulmonary shunting by increasing cardiac output (see Table 9–3).

Pulmonary Capillary Oxygen Content

As stated earlier, the pulmonary capillary oxygen content is considered a theoretical entity; its mathematical calculation is based on theoretical concepts. The calculation of the pulmonary capillary oxygen content depends in part on the calculation of a mean alveolar oxygen tension. This value represents a hypothetical average alveolar oxygen tension and may not represent the true alveolar oxygen tension of any particular alveolus. Chapter 7 discusses the fact that alveolar oxygen tensions vary throughout the lung and therefore it is convenient to deal mathematically with the concept of an *ideal alveolar oxygen tension.*

Ideal Alveolar Gas Equation

The calculation of an ideal alveolar oxygen tension is obtained from the ideal alveolar gas equation.[250] This equation corrects for changes in oxygen tension due to the fact that the respiratory exchange ratio is less than 1.0 (approximately 0.8 — see Chapters 5 and 6). This means that less carbon dioxide is transferred into the alveoli than the amount of oxygen removed from the alveoli. The arterial carbon dioxide tension can be used to replace the alveolar carbon dioxide tension since it is a very close approximation. An approximation of the ideal alveolar gas equation is:

$$P_{A_{O_2}} = [P_B - P_{H_2O}]F_{I_{O_2}} - \frac{P_{a_{CO_2}}}{0.8} \tag{15}$$

Under clinical circumstances where the arterial carbon dioxide tension is less than 60 mm Hg, and especially when oxygen therapy is being administered, it is acceptable to use an even more simplified version of the alveolar gas equation:[2]

$$P_{A_{O_2}} = [P_B - P_{H_2O}]F_{I_{O_2}} - P_{a_{CO_2}} \tag{16}$$

The Modified Clinical Shunt Equation

When arterial oxygen tension is greater than 150 mm Hg, the arterial hemoglobin may be considered fully saturated with oxygen. In this situation it is logical to assume that the hemoglobin in the portion of the cardiac output exchanging perfectly ($\dot{Q}C$) is also 100% saturated since it must always have as high or higher oxygen content than arterial blood. Therefore, the only difference in oxygen content between pulmonary capillary blood and arterial blood exists in the dissolved form. Under these limited clinical conditions a modified form of the clinical shunt equation may be written:

$$\frac{\dot{Q}s}{\dot{Q}T} = \frac{[P_{A_{O_2}} - P_{a_{O_2}}][0.003]}{[C_{a_{O_2}} - C\bar{v}_{O_2}] + [P_{A_{O_2}} - P_{a_{O_2}}][0.003]} \tag{17}$$

In most circumstances in which this modified form is used, the arterial-mixed venous oxygen content difference is usually assumed; that is, the clinical condition under which the application of this form of the equation is reasonable is one in which the cardiovascular reserve may be considered adequate and therefore the arterial to venous oxygen content is within normal limits. It has been noted that in resting, healthy human volunteers, the normal A-V content difference ranges between 4.5 and 6.0 vol%.[251,252] However, it has been recently documented that most critically ill, and especially those patients receiving ventilator support, who are maintaining cardiovascular stability have arterial to venous oxygen content differences below normal, i.e., ranging between 2.5 and 4.5 vol%.[253] On this basis an assumed value of 3.5 vol% is more representative in the critically ill patient fulfilling the above criteria.

Alveolar to Arterial Oxygen Gradients

The oxygen content difference in the numerator of equation (17) is based on the difference between oxygen tensions in the end pulmonary capillary blood (PA_{O_2}) and in arterial blood (Pa_{O_2}). This difference in oxygen dissolved in the blood is clinically referred to as the *alveolar to arterial oxygen tension gradient.* In clinical circumstances in which the cardiovascular reserve and the arterial-venous oxygen content difference may be reasonably assumed, and the arterial oxygen tension is greater than 150 mm Hg, the $A - aD_{O_2}$ may be used clinically to reflect intrapulmonary shunting. It should be noted that it is only under these limited clinical conditions that the alveolar to arterial oxygen tension gradient reflects a clinically useful, reliable measurement.

In summary, there are essentially two ways of quantitating the degree of intrapulmonary shunting: (1) alveolar to arterial oxygen tension differences and (2) shunt ratios. The measurement of $A - a$ differences is limited to giving only a qualitative estimate of the degree of intrapulmonary shunting. It will vary with changes in inspired oxygen concentrations as well as with changes in cardiovascular status. On the other hand, the calculation of the shunt ratio can give both a measure of the degree of intrapulmonary shunting and the patient's cardiovascular response to that level of intrapulmonary shunting. The additional clinical information obtained by the shunt measurement in acute respiratory care emphasizes the importance of understanding the significance of and technique for making pulmonary artery blood samples clinically available.

20 / Pulmonary Artery Blood Gases

THE PLACEMENT of pulmonary artery catheters for monitoring left ventricular hemodynamic function in critically ill patients has become accepted clinical practice over the past five years.[254-258] Although the initial purpose for developing such catheters and their early application dealt primarily with the need to monitor left heart filling pressures, these catheters also provide access to pulmonary artery blood for blood gas measurement. Repeated clinical observations determined that when these pulmonary artery blood gases are used in conjunction with arterial blood gas measurements, the results frequently clarify the cardiopulmonary status and allow appropriate therapeutic procedures to be instituted and monitored.[259, 260] The clinical importance of pulmonary artery blood gases is now appreciated in the care of the critically ill patient and the need for such measurements can be considered justification for placement of a pulmonary artery catheter.

Pulmonary Artery Catheters

Development of the Swan-Ganz, balloon-tipped catheter has made right heart and pulmonary artery catheterization technically feasible and relatively safe to perform at the bedside of the patient in intensive care.[261] The basic double-channel catheter has a fluid channel which opens at the distal tip and a second air channel connected to a balloon located close to the end of the catheter. The balloon may be repeatedly inflated and deflated with small amounts of air.

Placement

The catheter is introduced into the systemic venous system by either a surgical cut down over the antecubital fossa or percutaneously via either the subclavian or the internal jugular vein. The catheter is advanced with the balloon deflated until it lies within the chest cavity. The balloon is then appropriately inflated and further advanced, allowing the blood flow to carry the balloon tip in a manner similar to an embolus. In essence, the blood flow "carries" the tip of the catheter through the right ventricle and pulmonic valve into the pulmonary artery. Prior to introduction of the catheter, the fluid channel is filled with heparinized saline and connected to a pressure transducer allow-

227

ing for instantaneous display of the various pressure patterns on an os-cilloscope (cathode ray tube projection on a phosphorescent screen). A continuous ECG recording is essential for careful monitoring during advancement of the catheter. It is not unusual for the catheter tip to cause a few ventricular premature contractions as it passes through the right ventricle. Occasionally a severe ventricular arrhythmia will occur, necessitating immediate removal of the catheter from the right ventricle. The balloon should not be deflated with the tip of the catheter in the right ventricle.

Pressure Patterns

Figure 20–1 illustrates the pressure patterns displayed as the catheter tip traverses the right atrium, right ventricle, and main pulmonary artery and eventually lodges in a pulmonary artery branch in a wedge position.

Wedge Position

The catheter tip is positioned so that the inflated balloon completely occludes blood flow through a branch of the pulmonary artery. With the balloon deflated there must be free flow of pulmonary artery blood around the tip of the catheter. Inflation of the balloon should be kept to a minimum since blood flow to a significant portion of lung is obstructed while the balloon is occluding the vessel. It is also possible for the tip of the catheter to advance (migrate outward) after the catheter is initially positioned. In some circumstances this can result in an occlusion of the arterial branch even with the balloon deflated. This complication can be avoided by continuous monitoring of the pulmonary artery pressure pattern so that if a dampened pressure reading is observed, the catheter may be retracted and repositioned until a satisfactory pulmonary artery pressure pattern is obtained. Before this maneuver is attempted the catheter channel should be vigorously irrigated and the integrity of the pressure transducers thoroughly evaluated.

With the balloon properly inflated, the pressure reading just beyond the catheter tip will reflect back pressure through the pulmonary circulation. These "wedged" pressure readings relate to the filling pressure of the left ventricle in a manner similar to the way central venous pressure readings relate to right ventricular filling pressures. This is of obvious clinical importance in those patients who have normal right heart function with primary left heart dysfunction.

With the balloon deflated the pressure reading will represent the phasic (systolic/diastolic) pulmonary artery pressures. Under these circumstances a blood sample properly drawn through the fluid chan-

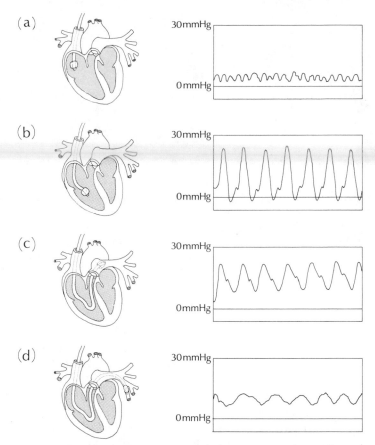

Fig 20–1.—Typical pressure patterns as the tip of the Swan-Ganz catheter traverses the right heart and pulmonary artery. **a,** right atrial pressure; **b,** right ventricular pressure—note that diastolic pressure is zero baseline or below; **c,** pulmonary artery pressure—note that diastolic pressure is significantly above zero baseline; **d,** pulmonary wedge pressure—catheter tip senses only pulmonary capillary back pressure since balloon obstructs arterial flow. Deflation of the balloon should result in immediate return of the pulmonary artery pressure pattern (see text).

nel (see Chapter 14) is obviously pulmonary artery blood and will have a true mixed venous oxygen tension and content.

Thermodilution Cardiac Output Measurements

A triple-channel pulmonary artery catheter contains a second fluid-filled channel that ends approximately 30 cm from the tip of the cathe-

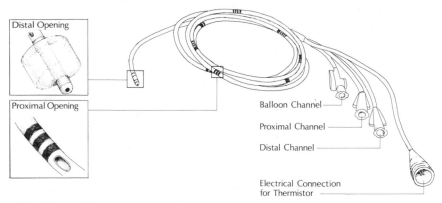

Fig 20–2.—The four-channel pulmonary artery catheter. The distal channel and balloon channel comprise the basic two-channel catheter. Addition of the proximal channel that opens in the right atrium results in the triple-channel catheter, usually 7 French in diameter. Addition of the thermistor channel results in the four-channel catheter used for thermodilution cardiac output measurements, usually 7 French in diameter.

ter. This opening is designed to lie in the right atrium or superior vena cava and is used as a central venous pressure monitor.

The four-channel pulmonary artery catheter (Fig 20–2) has a thermistor located near the tip of the catheter and an electrical circuit leading from the thermistor to a calculator. A known quantity of cold solution may be injected into the channel whose outlet is in the area of the right atrium. The temperature of this solution (usually 10 ml of iced 5% dextrose and water) and the patient's rectal temperature are measured. The injected solution mixes with blood in the right ventricle and is ejected into the pulmonary artery over several ventricular contractions. The net effect of this mixing is to temporarily decrease the temperature of the blood passing through the pulmonary artery during this short interval of time. The temperature change is measured by the thermistor at the end of the catheter.[264] Cardiac output is then calculated from knowing the amount of cold injected and the average concentration of cold during the time required for total ejection of the cold solution from the right ventricle.[265, 266] In reality, this technique represents an expression of the Fick equation used classically in determining cardiac output ($\dot{Q}T$).[262] The quantity of cold injected represents the solute replacing the oxygen consumption ($\dot{V}O_2$) and the average measured temperature change of the blood replaces the arterial-mixed venous oxygen content difference ($Ca_{O_2} - C\bar{v}_{O_2}$) in the Fick equation. In all Swan-Ganz catheters, the fluid-filled channel that empties at the tip of the catheter (the distal channel) may be used to obtain pulmonary artery blood samples.

Central Venous Blood Gases

The superior and inferior vena cava represent a composite of several different organ systems. However, the coronary blood flow has an extremely high degree of oxygen extraction and is not represented by a blood sample taken from either vena cava because the coronary sinus empties directly into the right atrium. Blood taken from catheters with the tip placed in the right atrium shows tremendous variation from sample to sample because of channeling of blood flow through the atrium from the various venous sources. Samples from a catheter tip in the right ventricle are also highly variable and the catheter tip acts as a source of ventricular ectopic activity.[9]

In healthy human subjects at rest, venous samples taken simultaneously from a catheter in the superior vena cava and pulmonary artery give reasonably close values. In critically ill patients this close relationship does not exist; however, an excellent correlation between superior vena cava and pulmonary artery blood can be demonstrated in the critically ill patient as blood flow to critical organ systems becomes a priority. The general statement may be made that in the critically ill patient with a stable cardiovascular state and good peripheral perfusion, oxygen tensions in superior vena cava blood are a reliable reflection of those in pulmonary artery blood.[253]

Mixed Venous Oxygen Measurements

A true mixed venous oxygen tension may be measured only in the outflow tract of the right ventricle—the pulmonary artery. Several studies of pulmonary artery blood from healthy human volunteers have revealed a mixed venous oxygen tension of 40 mm Hg and an average arterial-venous oxygen content difference of approximately 5 vol%. These same subjects had normal systemic arterial blood gases, with their pulmonary artery blood revealing a carbon dioxide tension range of 44–46 mm Hg and a pH range of 7.34–7.36.

In critically ill patients these traditional values relating to normal healthy volunteers can no longer be applied. It has been repeatedly demonstrated that critically ill patients with adequate cardiovascular reserves increase their cardiac output above their normal resting value in response to their increased physiologic demands. These cardiac output values are routinely expressed as a *cardiac index* (L/min/sq m body surface area), thus accounting for differences in size. The net effect is a decrease in the amount of oxygen extracted from each aliquot of blood (a decreased arterial-venous oxygen content difference). The critically ill patient who begins to decompensate will often have a theoretically normal cardiac output (cardiac index) for a time period before complete decompensation occurs. Simultaneously there is an increased arterial-venous oxygen extraction and a decreased mixed venous oxygen tension. These findings are often observed before significant changes in arterial oxygen tension occur.

Arterial-Venous Oxygen Content Difference

Table 20–1 lists reference values relating to pulmonary artery blood gas samples and the derived values. The clinical application of these values also requires a simultaneous measurement of an arterial blood gas. These values should be considered only as guidelines and they assume a normal oxygen-carrying capacity, clinical evidence of adequate peripheral perfusion, adequate alveolar ventilation, and normal acid-base status with either the patient breathing spontaneously or being supported on the ventilator.[263]

Once other factors such as severe anemia, lack of peripheral perfusion, severe hypercarbia, and acidemia are superimposed, these guidelines begin to lose their clinical usefulness. These physiologic

TABLE 20–1.—PREDICTED BLOOD GAS VALUES IN HEALTH
AND DISEASE FOR PULMONARY ARTERY BLOOD

CONDITION	$P\bar{v}_{O_2}$		% Hb SAT.		$[Ca_{O_2} - C\bar{v}_{O_2}]$ (vol%)	
	RANGE	AVERAGE	RANGE	AVERAGE	RANGE	AVERAGE
Healthy resting human volunteer	37–43	40	70–76	75	4.5–6.0	5.0
Critically ill patient, cardiovascular reserves excellent	35–40	37	68–75	70	2.5–4.5	3.5
Critically ill patient, cardiovascular stable, limited cardiovascular reserves	30–35	32	56–68	60	4.5–6.0	5.0
Critically ill patient, cardiovascular decompensation	< 30	< 30	< 56	< 56	> 6.0	> 6.0

measurements should be used as early warning indicators of impending or early cardiovascular decompensation. Their clinical value lies in the fact that changes in venous (pulmonary artery) blood gases often occur earlier than changes in routine arterial blood gases, therefore allowing for the initiation of corrective therapeutic maneuvers reversing the pathophysiology at an earlier stage.

Intrapulmonary Shunting versus Myocardial Failure

In the critically ill patient with a significant hypoxemia, ascertaining the exact physiologic defect and defining whether the cardiac or pulmonary systems or both are implicated often present a diagnostic challenge. Careful clinical evaluation, including a detailed history and physical examination, routine laboratory studies, chest x-ray, and blood work, often does not give the answer. In the critically ill patient the question of a large primary intrapulmonary shunt versus primary myocardial dysfunction becomes paramount since it dictates the emphasis of treatment. If it is an intrapulmonary shunt, such therapies as mobilization of secretions, the use of antimicrobial agents to eradicate infection or PEEP may be pertinent. If it is myocardial dysfunction, alteration of vascular volume to vascular space relationships or the institution of myocardial inotropic agents may become important.

In Chapter 19 the shunt equation was derived and it was demonstrated to be an effective tool for assessing the cause of hypoxemia since it allows for analysis of both intrapulmonary shunting and the cardiac output, the major effective compensation for shunting.

$$\frac{\dot{Q}s}{\dot{Q}T} = \frac{[Cc_{O_2} - Ca_{O_2}]}{[Ca_{O_2} - C\bar{v}_{O_2}] + [Cc_{O_2} - Ca_{O_2}]}$$

The theoretical end pulmonary oxygen content minus the arterial oxygen content $[Cc_{O_2} - Ca_{O_2}]$ represents an assessment of the intrapulmonary shunting. The arterial oxygen content minus the mixed venous oxygen content difference $[Ca_{O_2} - C\bar{v}_{O_2}]$ represents an assessment of the cardiovascular response to the intrapulmonary shunt (cardiac output). This becomes obvious when the arterial-mixed venous oxygen content difference is considered in the context of the Fick equation:

$$\dot{Q}T = \frac{\dot{V}O_2}{[Ca_{O_2} - C\bar{v}_{O_2}]}$$
$$\dot{V}O_2 = [\dot{Q}T][Ca_{O_2} - C\bar{v}_{O_2}]$$

TABLE 20-2.—RELATIONSHIP OF CARDIAC OUTPUT TO
OXYGEN EXTRACTION

CONDITION	OXYGEN CONSUMPTION (cc/min)	CARDIAC OUTPUT ($\dot{Q}T$) (L/min)	OXYGEN EXTRACTION $(Ca_{O_2} - C\bar{v}_{O_2})$ [vol% (cc/L)]
Normal cardiac output	250	5	5 (50)
Increased cardiac output	250	10	2.5 (25)
Decreased cardiac output	250	2.5	10 (100)

Under conditions in which the oxygen consumption ($\dot{V}O_2$) remains constant, changes in cardiac output ($\dot{Q}T$) can be directly related to changes in arterial-mixed venous oxygen content differences ($Ca_{O_2} - C\bar{v}_{O_2}$). In other words, as cardiac output increases under these circumstances, oxygen extraction per unit volume of blood decreases (Table 20-2).

In critically ill patients who are controlled on the ventilator (no change in muscle work) with a stable temperature, it is often clinically reasonable to assume a constant oxygen consumption. Therefore, in these patients changes in arterial-mixed venous oxygen content differences directly reflect changes in cardiac output. This has clinical significance since for any level of intrapulmonary shunting, the arterial oxygen tension will be dependent in part upon the cardiac output.[252] As the cardiac output decreases, the arterial oxygen tension decreases even though the intrapulmonary shunt remains unchanged (Table 20-3).

Summary

The development of the balloon-tipped pulmonary artery catheter has made pulmonary artery measurements available at the bedside of the critically ill patient. Besides hemodynamic monitoring, blood gas measurements of true mixed venous blood values, in con-

TABLE 20-3.—COMPARISON EFFECT OF CARDIAC OUTPUT ON
THE ARTERIAL OXYGEN TENSION

$\dot{Q}s/\dot{Q}T$ (%)	$\dot{V}O_2$ (cc)	$\dot{Q}T$ (L/min)	$[Ca_{O_2} - C\bar{v}_{O_2}]$ (vol%)	Pa_{O_2} (mm Hg)
25	250	10	2.5	127
25	250	5	5.0	84
25	250	2.5	10.0	55

PA_{O_2} = 355 mm Hg, FI_{O_2} = 50%, Hb = 15 gm %, Cc_{O_2} = 21.17 vol%.

junction with arterial blood gas values, have allowed the clinician to more clearly identify the cardiopulmonary pathophysiology. This has further reinforced the interdependence of the two systems. The next step in sophistication depends on the further development of noninvasive techniques which can give the same information.

Case Studies in the Clinical Application of Blood Gas Measurement

THIS SECTION contains brief presentations of cases treated in the Respiratory Intensive Care area of Northwestern Memorial Hospital. Each case illustrates a critical point concerning the clinical application of blood gas analysis to supportive care. Reference to portions of the text containing appropriate discussions is made at the end of each case.

This section is meant for self-testing comprehension of the material presented in the text. By no means do these cases represent all possible problems; rather, they represent "typical" or "usual" clinical problems in respiratory care.

Case 1

A 17-year-old diabetic entered the emergency room with Kussmaul breathing and irregular pulse.

Room air blood gases:

pH	7.05	HCO_3^-	5 mEq/L
Pco_2	12 mm Hg	BE	−30 mEq/L
Po_2	108 mm Hg		

Interpretation: Severe partly compensated metabolic acidosis without hypoxemia.

Glucose and insulin, intravenously, were immediately started. However, it was felt that the severe acidosis was not being tolerated by the cardiovascular system, and the physician elected to rapidly restore the pH to the 7.20 range.

This was a 103-pound girl. Before going on, calculate the amount of sodium bicarbonate you would have given.

$$103 \text{ pounds} = 47 \text{ kg}$$
$$\frac{1}{3} \times 47 = 16 \text{ L}$$
$$30 \times 16 = 480 \text{ mEq total deficit}$$

Because it was considered desirable to partly correct the acidosis, one half was given; i.e., a 240 mEq intravenous push in 15 minutes. Ten minutes later the blood gases were:

pH	7.27	HCO_3^-	11 mEq/L
P_{CO_2}	25 mm Hg	BE	-14 mEq/L
P_{O_2}	92 mm Hg		

Case 2

A 66-year-old woman with a history of chronic obstructive pulmonary disease entered the emergency room in obvious pulmonary edema.

Room air blood gases:

pH	7.10	HCO_3^-	8 mEq/L	BP	60/?
P_{CO_2}	25 mm Hg	BE	-20 mEq/L	P	140/min, thready
P_{O_2}	40 mm Hg	S_{O_2}	52%		

Interpretation: Partly compensated metabolic acidosis with severe hypoxemia. (Hypoxia must be assumed when acidemia and hypoxemia coexist.)

The patient received IPPB with high oxygen concentration and 50% ethyl alcohol in the nebulizer. After 10 minutes:

pH	7.38	HCO_3^-	16 mEq/L	BP	100/40
P_{CO_2}	28 mm Hg	BE	-7 mEq/L	P	140/min, strong
P_{O_2}	110 mm Hg	S_{O_2}	99%		

The lactic acidosis was reversed.

Case 3

A 17-year-old girl with severe kyphoscoliosis entered the hospital with pneumonia.

$F_{I_{O_2}}$ 40%:

pH	7.37	HCO_3^-	14 mEq/L

Pco$_2$	25 mm Hg	BE	−7 mEq/L
Po$_2$	70 mm Hg	So$_2$	93%

Interpretation: Chronic alveolar hyperventilation with uncorrected hypoxemia.

The patient was on fluids intravenously for three days. The fever and the rales disappeared with antibiotic therapy. However, she began to complain of weakness and difficulty in breathing.

Room air blood gases:

pH	7.53	HCO$_3^-$	25 mEq/L
Pco$_2$	31 mm Hg	BE	+4 mEq/L
Po$_2$	62 mm Hg		

Interpretation: In light of this girl's previous gases, this must be interpreted as uncompensated metabolic alkalosis.

Serum electrolytes revealed a hypokalemia. After proper KCl replacement, the patient had no complaints.

Room air blood gases:

pH	7.41	HCO$_3^-$	16 mEq/L
Pco$_2$	27 mm Hg	BE	−6 mEq/L
Po$_2$	65 mm Hg		

Interpretation: Her normal state of chronic alveolar hyperventilation with mild hypoxemia.

Case 4

A 47-year-old man collapsed on the street and was brought to the emergency room. On admission he was blue, without palpable pulse, and was making agonal respiratory movements. The airway was cleared, ventilation established with 100% oxygen and closed-chest cardiac massage instituted. Within 20 seconds there was a palpable pulse and skin color improved. The patient became alert and uncooperative within 2 minutes.

Twenty minutes following the successful resuscitation, blood gas samples were drawn. The patient had received 100 mEq of sodium bicarbonate and 300 ml of 5% dextrose/water intravenously. What would you expect his blood gases to be on 40% oxygen?

pH	7.51	HCO_3^-	27 mEq/L
PCO_2	35 mm Hg	BE	+5 mEq/L
PO_2	62 mm Hg		

Interpretation: Uncompensated metabolic alkalosis with uncorrected hypoxemia. This patient may manifest alveolar hyperventilation without oxygen therapy. The metabolic alkalosis is expected.

Case 5

A 54-year-old woman with a 10-year history of "heart failure" was taking diuretics regularly. She had a "chest cold" the last week and experienced progressive shortness of breath.

Room air blood gases:

pH	7.54	HCO_3^-	22 mEq/L	VT	600 ml	BP	160/100
PCO_2	26 mm Hg	BE	+2 mEq/L	RR	25/min	P	110/min
PO_2	48 mm Hg	SO_2	89%	MV	15 L	T	100°F

Interpretation: Acute alveolar hyperventilation with moderate hypoxemia. Hypoxia probably is not present because the cardiovascular system appears intact. This is probably a shunt-producing cardiopulmonary disease because the minute volume is reflected in the alveolar ventilation. The alveolar hyperventilation is most likely due to the hypoxemia. Oxygen therapy is indicated.

FI_{O_2} 40%:

pH	7.48	HCO_3^-	23 mEq/L	VT	500 ml	BP	140/90
PCO_2	31 mm Hg	BE	+1 mEq/L	RR	20/min	P	100/min
PO_2	55 mm Hg	SO_2	91%	MV	10 L	T	100°F

This patient had a right pleural effusion causing atelectasis and shunting. Three liters of fluid were removed. The patient received IPPB, and the next day:

FI_{O_2} 40%:

pH	7.42	HCO₃⁻	22 mEq/L	VT	400 ml	BP	120/80

pH 7.42 HCO_3^- 22 mEq/L VT 400 ml BP 120/80
PCO_2 36 mm Hg BE −1 mEq/L RR 12/min P 90/min
PO_2 90 mm Hg SO_2 97% MV 4.8 L T 99°F

Interpretation: Normal ventilatory status with corrected hypoxemia.

Case 6

A 47-year-old woman is in the recovery room for 3 hours after gallbladder removal. She has been receiving 40% FI_{O_2} and a blood gas is drawn to assess the oxygen therapy.

pH 7.44 Sat 98% BP 130/90
PCO_2 30 mm Hg Hb 13.2 gm% P 95, regular
PO_2 121 mm Hg BE −2 mEq/L RR 20/min
VT 350 ml

The physician decides to decrease FI_{O_2} to 30% and requests a blood gas measurement to be obtained in 30 minutes. One-half hour later there is no apparent clinical change and the blood gases and vital signs are repeated:

pH 7.41 Sat 96% BP 130/90
PCO_2 10 mm Hg Hb 7.4 gm% P 95, regular
PO_2 148 mm Hg BE −17 mEq/L RR 22/min
VT 350 ml

A technical error is suspected—repeat measurements on 30% FI_{O_2} reveal:

pH 7.45 Sat 96%
PCO_2 31 mm Hg Hb 13.1 gm%
PO_2 87 mm Hg BE −2 mEq/L

What was the most likely technical error?

A delay in running the sample would decrease the PO_2; exposure to room air would result in an increased pH for the PCO_2 drop; too much sodium heparin could explain these erroneous results.

Case 7

A 53-year-old man enters the coronary care unit with chest pain and a presumptive diagnosis of acute myocardial infarction. Arterial blood gases are drawn to assess the need for oxygen therapy. The patient is uncooperative and there is difficulty obtaining the radial artery sample. Vital signs are stable except for occasional PVCs. The patient is breathing room air.

pH	7.57	BP	110/70
PCO_2	24 mm Hg	P	90
PO_2	140 mm Hg	RR	20/min
		V_T	400 ml

Repeat sample shows:

pH	7.49
PCO_2	35 mm Hg
PO_2	75 mm Hg

What is the most probable explanation?

Case 8

A 47-year-old man without previous illness entered the coronary care unit with an ECG diagnosis of "inferior wall infarct" and severe chest pain. He had received morphine in the emergency room. Cardiac monitor showed numerous PVCs.

Room air blood gases:

pH	7.51	HCO_3^-	23 mEq/L	BP	100/60
PCO_2	29 mm Hg	BE	0 mEq/L	P	120/min, irregular
PO_2	64 mm Hg	SO_2	94%	RR	22/min

Interpretation: Acute alveolar hyperventilation with mild hypoxemia.

FI_{O_2} 40%:

pH	7.47	HCO_3^-	24 mEq/L	BP	110/60
PCO_2	32 mm Hg	BE	0 mEq/L	P	110/min, regular
PO_2	66 mm Hg	SO_2	94%	RR	22/min

The oxygen therapy decreased myocardial and ventilatory demand. The arrhythmia disappeared, the chest pain diminished, and the patient felt better.

Note: Oxygen therapy is not the suggested method for treating arrhythmia. However, it is common to have arrhythmia diminish or disappear when oxygen is properly applied.

Case 9

A 63-year-old man is admitted for elective knee surgery. Blood gases were obtained as part of the preoperative work-up. The results obtained on room air were:

pH	7.36	SO_2	74%	P	80, regular
PCO_2	46 mm Hg	BE	0 mEq/L	RR	15/min
PO_2	41 mm Hg	BP	122/84	VT	450 ml

Interpretation: Technical error is suspected since there are no clinical signs of severe hypoxemia. The most likely cause is a venous sample.

Case 10

A 9-year-old boy with a history of allergic asthma had been audibly wheezing for one week. He had been placed on penicillin, plus oral bronchodilators, for one week. His mother stated he had not slept in two nights. The child was sitting and was using all accessory muscles to breathe. The wheezes could be heard from across the room.

Room air blood gases:

pH	7.41	HCO_3^-	15 mEq/L	VT	500 ml	BP	160/100
PCO_2	25 mm Hg	BE	−7 mEq/L	RR	30/min	P	130/min
PO_2	35 mm Hg	SO_2	62%	MV	15 L	T	101°F

Interpretation: Chronic alveolar hyperventilation with severe hypoxemia. Decreased oxygen content and work of breathing make tissue hypoxia a strong possibility. The cardiovascular system is working very hard. Even though this child is not in ventilatory failure, his cardiopulmonary reserve is marginal.

Epinephrine subcutaneously, IPPB with Isuprel, and intravenous fluids were started.

FI_{O_2} 40%:

pH	7.44	HCO_3^-	19 mEq/L	Vt	400 ml	BP	150/100
Pco_2	29 mm Hg	BE	−4 mEq/L	RR	20/min	P	130/min
Po_2	55 mm Hg	So_2	90%	MV	8 L		

The rise in pH despite the rise in Pco_2 suggests there had been lactic acidosis present that was corrected by oxygen therapy. Both ventilatory and oxygenation states were markedly improved.

Case 11

A 47-year-old woman had her gallbladder removed. On the second postoperative day she complained of chest pain.

Room air blood gases:

pH	7.45	HCO_3^-	17 mEq/L	Vt	500 ml	BP	130/70
Pco_2	25 mm Hg	BE	−5 mEq/L	RR	24/min	P	100/min
Po_2	58 mm Hg	So_2	95%	MV	12 L	T	100°F

Interpretation: Chronic alveolar hyperventilation with moderate hypoxemia. There is no evidence of deadspace disease. Remember, these are not uncommon blood gases on the second day after an upper abdominal procedure.

Atelectasis and pneumonia must be ruled out. There is little evidence to support the existence of pulmonary embolus. Oxygen therapy is indicated to reduce ventilatory and myocardial work.

Case 12

A 21-year-old woman in the third trimester of pregnancy fell on the ice and fractured her right forearm.

Room air blood gases:

pH	7.42	HCO_3^-	19 mEq/L	VT	500 ml
PCO_2	29 mm Hg	BE	−4 mEq/L	RR	16/min
PO_2	77 mm Hg	SO_2	96%	MV	8 L

Interpretation: Chronic alveolar hyperventilation with mild hypoxemia. These are normal for the third trimester of pregnancy. Oxygen therapy is *not* indicated.

Reference	*Page*
Chapter 17 Third-trimester pregnancy	205

Case 13

A 24-year-old woman entered the emergency room with a broken ankle. She appeared somewhat disoriented and confused.

Room air blood gases:

pH	7.55	HCO_3^-	23 mEq/L
PCO_2	27 mm Hg	BE	0 mEq/L
PO_2	105 mm Hg	SO_2	100%

Interpretation: Acute alveolar hyperventilation without hypoxemia. Little evidence of tissue hypoxia is present. This is most likely secondary to pain and anxiety.

Reference	*Page*
Chapter 17 Pain and anxiety	206

Case 14

A 67-year-old woman was admitted for uncontrolled rectal bleeding of several days' duration.

Room air blood gases:

pH	7.48	HCO_3^-	21 mEq/L	VT	450 ml	BP	160/90
PCO_2	28 mm Hg	BE	−1 mEq/L	RR	20/min	P	120/min
PO_2	95 mm Hg	SO_2	98%	MV	9 L		

Interpretation: Chronic alveolar hyperventilation without hypoxemia.

Hemoglobin content was 6 gm%. The chronic hyperventilation was due to the anemia. Control of the bleeding and transfusion resulted in normal blood gases and vital signs two days later.

Case 15

A 53-year-old fireman was overcome by smoke. In the emergency room with 50% oxygen by mask:

pH	7.58	HCO_3^-	21 mEq/L	VT	760 ml	BP 175/110
P_{CO_2}	23 mm Hg	BE	+1 mEq/L	RR	25/min	P 135/min
P_{O_2}	300 mm Hg	S_{O_2}	61%	MV	19 L	

Interpretation: Acute alveolar hyperventilation with excessively corrected hypoxemia; in fact, one wonders if hypoxemia would exist at room air. The cardiopulmonary system is working very hard.

The carboxyhemoglobin level was 40%; that is, 40% of the hemoglobin was saturated with carbon monoxide and unavailable to carry oxygen.

With high oxygen concentrations, the carboxyhemoglobin was reduced by 50% each hour.

Case 16

A 67-year-old woman was convalescent after a leg fracture. Four days after the fracture she had a sudden onset of severe chest pain and shortness of breath.

Room air blood gases:

pH	7.36	HCO_3^-	18 mEq/L	VT	720 ml	BP 130/90
P_{CO_2}	33 mm Hg	BE	−5 mEq/L	RR	25/min	P 100/min
P_{O_2}	55 mm Hg	S_{O_2}	88%	MV	18 L	T 99°F

Interpretation: Normal ventilatory status with moderate hypoxemia. The tremendous disparity between minute volume and alevolar ventilation suggests deadspace disease.

Pulmonary angiography revealed massive pulmonary emboli.

Case 17

A 27-year-old woman with pelvic inflammatory disease had chills, fever, and hypotension.

Room air blood gases:

pH	7.31	HCO_3^-	15 mEq/L	VT	430 ml	BP	60/0
P_{CO_2}	32 mm Hg	BE	−10 mEq/L	RR	35/min	P	130/min
P_{O_2}	55 mm Hg	S_{O_2}	86%	MV	15 L	T	103°F

Interpretation: Normal ventilatory status with moderate hypoxemia. The MV-alveolar ventilation disparity suggests deadspace disease—this may be due to tachypnea. The hypotension suggests hypoxia and may explain the base deficit (lactic acidosis).

Case 18

A 450-pound, 42-year-old woman entered the hospital for evaluation of gastrointestinal bypass procedure for obesity.

Baseline blood gases on room air:

pH	7.46	HCO_3^-	50 mEq/L
P_{CO_2}	72 mm Hg	BE	+20 mEq/L
P_{O_2}	53 mm Hg	S_{O_2}	89%

Interpretation: Chronic ventilatory failure with hypoxemia. This Pickwickian patient has a baseline of severe carbon dioxide retention. Oxygen therapy is contraindicated for the hypoxemia.

Case 19

A 76-year-old man with a long history of symptomatic chronic obstructive pulmonary disease entered the hospital with basilar pneumonia.

Room air blood gases:

pH	7.58	HCO_3^-	40 mEq/L
P_{CO_2}	45 mm Hg	BE	+15 mEq/L
P_{O_2}	38 mm Hg	S_{O_2}	83%

Interpretation: Uncompensated metabolic alkalosis with severe hypoxemia. But this diagnosis must be questioned! The *proper* interpretation is acute alveolar hyperventilation superimposed on chronic ventilatory failure. Careful oxygen therapy is indicated.

Case 20

A 76-year-old man with a long history of symptomatic chronic obstructive pulmonary disease entered the hospital with basilar pneumonia.

Room air blood gases:

pH	7.25	HCO_3^-	38 mEq/L
P_{CO_2}	90 mm Hg	BE	+5 mEq/L
P_{O_2}	34 mm Hg	S_{O_2}	58%

Interpretation: Acute ventilatory failure superimposed on chronic ventilatory failure. A trial of low-concentration oxygen is indicated.

Case 21

A 76-year-old woman with documented CO_2 retention secondary to severe COPD has been in the medical intensive care unit for 3 days with a diagnosis of acute bacterial pneumonitis. She has been stable for 24 hours with the following arterial blood gases and vital signs on a 28% Venturi mask:

pH	7.44	BP	135/95
P_{CO_2}	63 mm Hg	P	110, regular
P_{O_2}	52 mm Hg	RR	22/min
		V_T	250 ml

She is placed on a nasal cannula at 2 L/min flow and the blood gases and vital signs are repeated in one hour.

pH	7.36	BP	140/100
P_{CO_2}	75 mm Hg	P	105, regular
P_{O_2}	65 mm Hg	RR	24/min
		V_T	200 ml

Case 22

A 43-year-old man is admitted to the surgical intensive care unit from the operating room. He was in an auto accident 6 hours before and has undergone splenectomy, repair of liver lacerations, and repair of compound femoral fracture. Multiple transfusions were necessary and his chest is unstable bilaterally due to multiple rib fractures.

The anesthesiologist had difficulty maintaining perfusion during the procedure. Bilateral chest tubes are functioning adequately and bleeding continues in the chest. Multiple PVCs suggest the possibility of myocardial contusion.

Because of cardiovascular instability a Swan-Ganz catheter is placed. The patient is on 50% $F_{I_{O_2}}$ with controlled volume ventilation and acceptable Pa_{CO_2} and pH. Simultaneous radial artery and pulmonary samples are obtained and show:

	Radial arterial	Pulmonary artery
P_{O_2}	52 mm Hg	31 mm Hg
Hb	14 gm%	14 gm%
HbO_2	83%	50%
C_{O_2}	15.7 vol%	9.5 vol%

What is the man's A-V content difference and what is the significance of the finding?

Case 23

A 34-year-old woman entered the emergency room comatose. She was suspected of taking an overdose of an unknown drug.

Room air blood gases:

pH	7.15	HCO_3^-	28 mEq/L
P_{CO_2}	80 mm Hg	BE	0 mEq/L
P_{O_2}	60 mm Hg	S_{O_2}	80%

Interpretation: Acute ventilatory failure. Hypoxia must be assumed. Support of ventilation is immediately indicated.

Case 24

A 53-year-old man with myasthenia gravis was being maintained on a volume ventilator due to a cholinergic crisis, aspiration pneumonia, and withdrawal from all cholinergic medication. For several days he had been maintained on the same ventilatory parameters and his blood gases were:

pH	7.43	HCO_3^-	26 mEq/L	V_T	800 ml
P_{CO_2}	41 mm Hg	BE	+2 mEq/L	RR	14/min
P_{O_2}	74 mm Hg	S_{O_2}	95%	$F_{I_{O_2}}$	35%

The next morning his blood gases were:

pH	7.52	HCO_3^-	24 mEq/L	V_T	800 ml
P_{CO_2}	30 mm Hg	BE	+2 mEq/L	RR	14/min
P_{O_2}	45 mm Hg	S_{O_2}	86%	$F_{I_{O_2}}$	35%

Interpretation: Alveolar hyperventilation with respiratory alkalemia and uncorrected hypoxemia. This signals the acute collapse of a lung segment or lobe, producing an acute shunt plus increased air exchange in the ventilated lung.

Case 25

A 32-year-old woman has been hospitalized for 18 hours with a diagnosis of pelvic inflammatory disease. She suddenly complains of chills, becomes very febrile, and is peripherally cold and clammy. She becomes disoriented and is moved to medical intensive care with a diagnosis of septic shock.

Chest x-ray reveals diffuse infiltrates throughout both lung fields. The patient's breathing is rapid and labored. On 50% oxygen the arterial blood gases and vital signs are:

pH	7.32	BP	90/?
P_{CO_2}	34 mm Hg	P	140, regular
P_{O_2}	43 mm Hg	RR	36/min
Hb	12.5 gm%	V_T	400 ml

Due to the confusion as to the pulmonary versus cardiovascular components, a Swan-Ganz catheter is placed.

A-V oxygen content difference	2.7 vol%
Q_S/Q_T	52%

Is the hypoxemia due to septic shock? Might ARDS be entertained as a possibility?

Glossary

Symbols of Respiratory Physiology

GAS SYMBOLS
O_2 = oxygen
CO_2 = carbon dioxide
N_2 = nitrogen
H_2O = water

GENERAL PREFIXES
(full capitals only)
P = partial pressure (tension)
S = saturation of hemoglobin
C = content
V = ventilation
Q = cardiac output
F = fractional concentration in dry gas phase

SMALL CAPITALS
refer to the lung
A = alveolar gas
D = deadspace gas
$\overline{E}$ = mean expired gas
T = tidal gas

LOWERCASE LETTERS
refer to the blood
a = arterial
c = capillary
$\overline{v}$ = mixed venous

EXAMPLES
Pa_{O_2} = partial pressure of oxygen in arterial blood (arterial oxygen tension)
$S\overline{v}_{O_2}$ = mixed venous hemoglobin oxygen saturation
Cc_{O_2} = oxygen content in capillary blood
PA_{CO_2} = partial pressure of alveolar carbon dioxide (alveolar carbon dioxide tension)

Glossary

Absolute pressure—The total pressure above a vacuum; atmospheric pressure plus the gauge pressure.

Absolute shunt—The portion of the physiologic shunt secondary to anatomic and capillary shunting; the true physiologic shunt.

Acid—A substance capable of donating a hydrogen ion.

Acid, nonvolatile—An acid that cannot be eliminated by a gaseous route; e.g., lactic acid, keto acid.

Acid, volatile—An acid capable of undergoing a chemical reaction producing a gas; e.g., $H_2CO_3 \rightarrow CO_2 + H_2O$.

Acidemia—A pH below an acceptable level in arterial blood.

Acidity—The total amount of hydrogen ions in a solution measured by titration; not synonymous with free hydrogen ion concentration.

Acidosis—A pathophysiologic state where a significant base deficit is present.

Acute—Recent onset of a physiologic abnormality; usually refers to severity as well as suddenness of onset.

Aerobic metabolism—Use of metabolic pathways that utilize oxygen.

Affinity—The force with which atoms are held together; a natural attraction between atoms.

Air content—(1) Atmospheric (dry): O_2 21% (160 mm Hg), N_2 79% (600 mm Hg), CO_2 0.04% (0.3 mm Hg); (2) alveolar: O_2 14% (100 mm Hg), N_2 73% (573 mm Hg), CO_2 5.6% (40 mm Hg), water vapor 6.2% (47 mm Hg).

Airway—The normal path by which air travels from atmosphere to alveolus.

Alkalemia—A pH above an acceptable level in the arterial blood.

Alkalosis—A pathophysiologic state in which there is more than normal base present.

Alveolar-capillary membrane—Tissues separating alveolar gas from pulmonary blood: (1) alveolar epithelium, (2) interstitial tissue, (3) capillary endothelium.

Alveolar ventilation—That portion of the air movement in and out of the lungs that exchanges gas molecules with pulmonary blood; the effective ventilation. Alveolar hypoventilation is an arterial carbon dioxide tension above an acceptable limit, alveolar hyperventilation is an arterial carbon dioxide tension below an acceptable limit.

Alveolus—The gas exchange unit; the terminal air sac of the lung.

Anaerobic metabolism—Use of metabolic pathways that do not require oxygen; metabolite usually is lactic acid.

Anatomic shunt—Blood passing from right heart to left heart without entering pulmonary capillaries.

Anemia—A quantitative deficiency of the hemoglobin, usually involves a decrease in red blood cells.

Anion—A negatively charged ion.

Apex—The top of an organ; e.g., the lung apex is the top of the lung when the body is erect.

Apnea—Absence of breathing.

Arrhythmia—Any disturbance in the rhythm of the heartbeat.

Arrhythmia, ventricular—Abnormal heartbeat that originates in the ventricle.

Asphyxia—Death due to cessation of ventilation.

Aspiration—The entrance of foreign material into the tracheobronchial tree.

Atelectasis—Alveolar collapse.

Atmospheric pressure—The weight of the atmosphere; at sea level, 760 mm Hg, or 14.7 pounds per square inch.

Atrium—The two upper chambers of the heart; thin-walled, low-pressure structures very much affected by intrathoracic pressures.

Autonomic nervous system—The nervous system that is not under conscious control; composed of two antagonistic systems, called the sympathetic and parasympathetic systems.

Barometric pressure—The atmospheric pressure; the reading on a barometer.

Base—A substance that will accept hydrogen ions.

Base deficit—The number of milliequivalents per liter of bicarbonate below the normal base buffer level.

Base excess—The number of milliequivalents per liter of bicarbonate above the normal base buffer level.

Base, lung—The bottom of the lungs when the body is erect.

Bicarbonate ion—HCO_3^-; the major blood base.

Blood—The fluid that circulates in the vascular system; consists of formed elements (red blood cells) and fluid (plasma).

Blood gases—The gases dissolved in blood; primarily the measurement of dissolved oxygen and carbon dioxide pressures in blood. This text considers the blood gases Po_2, Pco_2, and pH.

Bradycardia—Abnormally slow heart rate.

Bradypnea—Abnormally slow ventilatory rate.

Bronchoconstriction—Narrowing of the bronchial lumen; usually refers to smooth muscle constriction; may be due to swelling of the mucosa.

Bronchodilatation—Widening of the bronchial lumen; usually refers to relaxation of the smooth muscle.

Bronchospasm—A continuous and severe degree of bronchoconstriction.

BTPS—Body temperature and pressure, saturated; 37°C at 760 mm Hg total pressure when P_{H_2O} is 47 mm Hg.

Buffer—A substance capable of neutralizing both acids and bases without appreciably changing the original pH.

Capacity, oxygen-carrying—See *Oxygen-carrying capacity*.

Capacity, pulmonary—A combination of two or more lung volumes; e.g., vital capacity.

Capillary—A thin-walled vessel connecting arterial and venous vessels; a blood vessel in which gas exchange occurs.

Carbon dioxide—The product of normal aerobic metabolism.

Carbon monoxide—A gas found in smoke and other combustion products that has great affinity for hemoglobin; in smoke inhalation, the substance that decreases the hemoglobin ability to carry oxygen.

Carbonic acid—The major blood acid; a volatile acid—H_2CO_3.

Carboxyhemoglobin—Hemoglobin in which the available oxygen-binding sites are occupied by carbon monoxide—HbCO.

Cardiac output—The quantity of blood pumped by the heart in one minute.

Cardiopulmonary system—The combined organ systems of the heart, blood vessels, and lungs.

Cardiovascular system—The organ system of the heart and blood vessels.

Cation—A positively charged ion.

Chemoreceptor—Special nervous tissue that sends afferent stimuli when the tissue undergoes chemical change; makes up the aortic and carotid bodies, which are stimulated primarily by decreased tissue Po_2 or decreased pH.

Chronic—A physiologic abnormality of long duration; usually refers to a compensated condition.

Clark electrode—The modern device for measuring oxygen tensions.

Controlled ventilation—The use of the ventilator in which the patient takes no physiologically meaningful active role in the ventilatory cycle.

Corrected barometric pressure—Barometric pressure minus 47 mm Hg (P_{H_2O} at 37°C).

Cyanosis—The blue coloration of skin and mucous membranes which may be caused by more than 5 gm% reduced hemoglobin.

Deadspace/tidal volume ratio (VD/VT) — Measurement of the portion of the tidal volume that does not exchange with blood.

Deadspace ventilation — Wasted ventilation. Physiologic deadspace is that portion of the ventilation that does not exchange with pulmonary blood; anatomic deadspace is the conducting air space; alveolar deadspace is alveolar air that does not exchange with blood.

Density — The relationship between the volume of a gas and its weight.

Diameter — The measurement of a straight line passing through the center of a circle.

Diaphragm — The muscular structure separating the thoracic from the abdominal cavity; the major muscle of ventilation.

Diastolic — The pressure at which audible blood pressure sounds disappear.

Diffusion — The movement of gas molecules from a point of higher pressure to one of lower pressure.

Dissociation — The state of a substance in solution in which the elements are separate and have net electric charges; the ionic state of a substance.

Dyspnea — The subjective complaint of difficult breathing.

Edema — Accumulation of fluid in tissue; swelling.

Effective ventilation — See *Alveolar ventilation*.

Electrocardiogram (ECG) — The written or visual reflection of the electrical activity of the heart.

Electrolytes — Ions in body fluids, essential for normal electric and osmolar phenomena to take place: sodium (Na^+), potassium (K^+), bicarbonate (HCO_3^-), and chloride (Cl^-) are the major electrolytes.

Electrons — Negatively charged subatomic particles. Electron activity is basic to all chemical reactions.

Element — A substance that cannot be made into a simpler substance; a substance of which one molecule is one atom.

Enzyme — A substance that speeds or slows a chemical reaction; a catalytic substance.

Equilibrium — The state of rest or balance due to the equal action of opposing forces.

Estimated shunt — Calculation of the physiologic shunt where the A-V oxygen content difference is assumed to be 3.5 vol%.

Eupnea — Normal breathing.

Exponential scale — The mathematical scale of the powers of base 10; a logarithmic scale.

External respiration — The exchange of gas molecules between blood and alveolar air.

FI_{O_2} — Fraction of inspired oxygen; the percentage of oxygen in inspired air.

Great vessels — In this text, the great veins (vena cavae, atria, pulmonary veins) and great artery (aorta) in the thorax.

Homeostasis — The condition in which the interrelationships of the physiologic systems are maintaining the normal state.

Hypercapnia — Above-normal carbon dioxide in blood.

Hypercarbia — See *Hypercapnia*.

Hyperkalemia — Above-normal serum potassium.

Hyperpnea — Tidal volumes above normal; deep breathing.

Hypertension — High blood pressure.

Hyperthermia — Body temperature above normal; fever.

Hyperventilation — Above-normal air movement in and out of the lungs.

Hypocapnea — Below-normal carbon dioxide in blood.

Hypocarbia — See *Hypocapnea.*

Hypokalemia — Below-normal serum potassium.

Hypopnea — Tidal volumes below normal; shallow breathing.

Hypotension — Low blood pressure; shock.

Hypothermia — Below-normal body temperature.

Hypoventilation — Below-normal air movement in and out of the lungs.

Hypovolemia — Below-normal blood volume.

Hypoxemia — Below-normal arterial oxygen tensions.

Hypoxia — The state of tissue oxygen deficiency.

Internal respiration — The exchange of gas molecules between blood and tissue.

Intrapleural pressure — Pressure (usually below atmospheric) within the pleural space; intrathoracic pressure.

Intrapulmonary pressure — The pressure within the lung; airway pressure.

Intrathoracic pressure — See *Intrapleural pressure.*

Ion — An element with a net electrical charge.

Ionic dissociation — See *Dissociation.*

Lactic acid — The product of anaerobic metabolic pathways; an abnormal blood acid.

Laminar flow — The flow of gas or liquid molecules in straight lines parallel to the sides of the conducting tube; a pattern of molecular flow in which friction between molecules is minimal; the molecular flow pattern of least resistance.

Lung capacities — A combination of two or more lung volumes.

Lung volumes — The four primary static volumes of the lung: tidal volume (VT), expiratory reserve volume (ERV), inspiratory reserve volume (IRV), residual volume (RV).

Mechanical support of ventilation — Providing part or all of the work of breathing by hand or machine; providing ventilation for a patient by mechanical means.

Metabolism — The cellular process, using biochemical pathways, in which energy is produced and expended; the essential biochemistry of the life process.

Metabolite — An end chemical product of metabolism; a waste product of metabolism, which must be excreted from the body.

Methemoglobin — See *Hemoglobin.*

Metric measurements — Some of the metric quantities and their equivalents used in this text are the following: 2.54 cm (centimeters) = 1 inch; 1 cm = 0.39 inch; 1 mm Hg (millimeter of mercury) = 1.37 cm H_2O; 1 L (liter) = 1,000 ml (milliliters); 3.79 L = 1 gallon; 1 gm (gram) = 0.03527 ounces avoirdupois; 1 mg (milligram) = 0.001 gm; 1 kg (kilogram) = 1,000 gm.

Microcirculation — The capillary system; the system of small blood vessels in which gas exchange takes place.

Minute volume — The air exchanged in the airway in one minute; tidal volume times respiratory rate.

Mnemonic — A word or words serving to assist the memory.

Myocardium — The heart muscle.

Oncotic pressure — The forces on one side of a semipermeable membrane that cause water to flow to that side; such factors as proteins in blood; the result of osmotic pressure.

Osmotic pressure — The force that a dissolved substance exerts on a semipermeable membrane which it cannot penetrate.

Oxygen affinity — The willingness to accept, or unwillingness to give up, oxygen molecules attached to hemoglobin.

Oxygen-carrying capacity — The total ability of blood to carry oxygen; the maximum possible oxygen content of blood.

Oxygen content — Total oxygen in blood; both oxyhemoglobin and dissolved oxygen.

Oxygen dissociation curve — A graph depicting the chemical dissociation of oxygen from hemoglobin in relation to varying plasma oxygen tensions.

Oxygen supply — The oxygen available to the tissues.

Partial pressure — The pressure exerted by one gas in a mixture of gases.

Pathophysiology — The abnormal changes of physiology induced by disease.

Perfusion — Blood flow through the microcirculatory system.

Permeability — The capacity of a membrane to allow molecules to pass through it.

pH — A logarithmic scale denoting hydrogen ion concentration.

Physiologic deadspace — That portion of the ventilation that does not exchange with pulmonary blood.

Physiologic shunt — That portion of the cardiac output that does not exchange with alveolar air.

Physiology — The science that deals with the functions of living organisms.

Plasma — Whole blood minus the red blood cells; the liquid portion of the blood.

Protons — Positively charged subatomic particles.

Radius — One half of the diameter.

Respiration — The exchange of gas molecules.

Respiratory failure — The inability of the lungs to meet the metabolic demands of the body; inadequate gas exchange.

Respiratory quotient — The ratio of the volume of CO_2 produced to the volume of O_2 consumed.

Sanz electrode — The modern pH electrode.

Semipermeable — Permeable to some substances and not to others.

Serum — The portion of whole blood that remains in the liquid state after clotting has occurred.

Severinghaus electrode — The modern CO_2 electrode.

Shunt — Passage of blood from artery to vein without undergoing gas exchange. See *Absolute shunt; Anatomic shunt; Estimated shunt; Physiologic shunt.*

Solubility coefficient — The arithmetic factor representing the degree to which a substance will dissolve in solution under specified physical conditions.

Solution — The dispersing of a substance homogeneously throughout a liquid without undergoing chemical change.

Standard bicarbonate — The measurement of plasma bicarbonate at a P_{CO_2} of 40 mm Hg.

Systemic — Pertaining to or affecting the body as a whole.

Systolic — The highest pressure at which audible blood pressure sounds appear.

Tachycardia — Above-normal heart rate.

Tachypnea — Above-normal ventilatory rate.
Tension — The partial pressure of a gas.
Thorax — The upper part of the trunk, between the neck and the abdomen.
Tidal volume — The volume of air moved into or out of the lungs in any single breath.
Tissue — An aggregate of cells of like function.
Torr — Same as mm Hg.
Total ventilation — The air moving into or out of the lungs.
Trachea — The windpipe; the conducting tube from the larynx to the bronchi.
Turbulent flow — The flow of gas or liquid molecules in random fashion; a pattern of molecular flow in which friction is maximum; the molecular flow pattern of greatest resistance.
Venous admixture — Shunting due to perfusion in excess of ventilation; uneven distribution of ventilation; VA/Q inequality.
Venous return — The return of blood to the right heart; affected by intrathoracic pressure.
Ventilation — Movement of air into and out of the lungs; total ventilation. See *Alveolar ventilation; Controlled ventilation; Deadspace ventilation; Effective ventilation; Mechanical support of ventilation.*
Ventilation/perfusion inequality — See *Venous admixture.*
Ventilatory failure — The failure of the pulmonary system to meet the carbon dioxide metabolic demands of the body.
Vital capacity — A maximum expiration following a maximum inspiration.
Volatile — Pertaining to the property of changing from liquid to gas. See *Acid, volatile.*
Volumes percent — The number of milliliters of oxygen per 100 ml blood.
Water vapor — Water in the gas phase.
Water vapor pressure — The partial pressure exerted by the water vapor present in a gas.

REFERENCES

GENERAL TEXTBOOKS
1. Bates, D. V., and Christie, R. V.: *Respiratory Function in Disease* (2d ed.; Philadelphia: W. B. Saunders Co., 1971).
2. Bendixen, H. H., *et al.: Respiratory Care* (St. Louis: C. V. Mosby Co., 1965).
3. Comroe, J. H., Jr.: *Physiology of Respiration* (2d ed.; Chicago: Year Book Medical Publishers, Inc., 1971).
4. Comroe, J. H., Jr., *et al.: The Lung: Clinical Physiology and Pulmonary Function Tests* (2d ed.; Chicago: Year Book Medical Publishers, Inc., 1962).
5. Cotes, J. E.: *Lung Function: Assessment and Application in Medicine* (3d ed.; Philadelphia: J. B. Lippincott Co., 1975).
6. Davenport, H. W.: *ABC of Acid-Base Chemistry* (6th ed.; Chicago: The University of Chicago Press, 1974).
7. Egan, D. F.: *Fundamentals of Respiratory Therapy* (2d ed.; St. Louis: C. V. Mosby Co., 1973).
8. Filley, G. F.: *Acid-Base and Blood Gas Regulation* (2d ed.; Philadelphia: Lea & Febiger, 1971).
9. Guyton, A. C.: *Textbook of Medical Physiology* (4th ed.; Philadelphia: W. B. Saunders Co., 1971).

10. Nunn, J. F.: *Applied Respiratory Physiology: With Special Reference to Anaesthesia* (New York: Butterworth & Co., Ltd., 1969).
11. Shapiro, B. A., Harrison, R. A., and Trout, C. A.: *Clinical Application of Respiratory Care* (Chicago: Year Book Medical Publishers, Inc., 1975).
12. West, J. B.: *Ventilation/Blood Flow and Gas Exchange* (2d ed.; Philadelphia: F. A. Davis Co., 1970).
13. Wintrobe, M. M., *et al.* (eds.): *Principles of Internal Medicine* (6th ed.; New York: McGraw-Hill Book Co., 1970).

SELECTED REFERENCES

14. Radford, E. P., Jr.: The Physics of Gases, in *The Handbook of Physiology, Respiration*, vol. 1 (Washington, D.C.: American Physiological Society, 1964).
15. Perutz, M. F.: Structure and Function of Haemoglobin, Federation of European Biochemical Societies, 1st Meeting, London, 1964, p. 143–44.
16. Roughton, F. J. W.: Transport of Oxygen and Carbon Dioxide, in *The Handbook of Physiology, Respiration*, vol. 1 (Washington, D.C.: American Physiological Society, 1964).
17. Perutz, M. F.: Stereochemistry of cooperative effects in haemoglobin, Nature 228:726, 1970.
18. Rossi, L., and Roughton, F. J. W.: The effect of carbamino-Hb compounds on the buffer power of human blood at 37°C., J. Physiol. (Lond.) 167:15, 1963.
19. Chanutin, A., and Curnish, R. R.: Effect of organic and inorganic phosphates on the oxygen equilibrium of human erythrocytes, Arch. Biochem. Biophys. 121:96, 1967.
20. Roughton, F. J. W., and Darling, R. C.: The effect of carbon monoxide on the oxyhemoglobin dissociation curve, Am. J. Physiol. 141:17, 1944.
21. Stewart, R. D., *et al.*: Experimental human exposure to carbon monoxide, Arch, Environ. Health 21:154, 1970.
22. Roughton, F. J. W.: The kinetics of haemoglobin. IV. The competition of carbon monoxide and oxygen for haemoglobin, Proc. Soc. Lond. *B* 115:473, 1934.
23. Darling, R. C., *et al.*: Some properties of human fetal and maternal blood, J. Clin. Invest. 20:739, 1941.
24. Bunn, H. F., and Jandl, J. H.: Control of hemoglobin function within the red cell, N. Engl. J. Med. 282:1414, 1970.
25. Oski, F. A., *et al.*: The effects of deoxygenation of adult and fetal hemoglobin on the synthesis of red cell 2,3-diphosphoglycerate and its in vivo consequences, J. Clin. Invest. 49:400, 1970.
26. Oski, F. A.: Red cell metabolism in the newborn infant. V. Glycolytic intermediates and glycolytic enzymes, Pediatrics 44:84, 1969.
27. Versmold, H., *et al.*: Blood oxygen affinity in infancy: The interaction of fetal and adult hemoglobin, oxygen capacity and red cell hydrogen ion and 2,3-diphosphoglycerate concentration, Respir. Physiol. 18:14, 1973.
28. Ferguson, J. K. W.: Carbamino compounds of CO_2 with haemoglobin and their role in the transport of CO_2, J. Physiol. (Lond.) 88:40, 1936.
29. Ferguson, J. K. W., and Roughton, F. J. W.: The chemical relationships and physiologic importance of carbamino compounds of CO_2 with haemoglobin, J. Physiol. (Lond.) 83:87, 1934.

30. Keilin, D., and Mann, T.: Activity of carbonic anhydrase within red blood corpuscles, Nature 148:493, 1941.
31. Bohr, Hasselbalch, and Krogh: Scand. Arch. Physiol. 16:402, 1904.
32. Christiansen, Douglas, and Haldane: J. Physiol. (Lond.) 48:244, 1914.
33. Cremer, M.: Z. Biol. 47:562, 1906.
34. Haber, F., and Klemensiewicz, Z.: Z. Physik. Chem. 67:385, 1909.
35. Borelius, G.: Ann. Physik. 45:929, 1914.
36. Gold, V.: *pH Measurements: Their Theory and Practice* (London: Methuen, 1958).
37. Bates, R. G.: *Electrometric pH Determinations* (John Wiley & Sons, Inc., 1954).
38. Blaedel, W. J., and Meloche, V. W.: *Elementary Quantitative Analysis Theory and Practice* (Harper & Row, 1963).
39. Adams, A. P., Morgan-Hughes, J. O., and Sykes, M. K.: pH and blood gas analysis, Anaesthesia 22:575, 1967.
40. Sanz, M. C.: Ultramicro methods and standardization of equipment, Clin. Chem. 3:406, 1957.
41. Anderson, O. S., *et al.*: A micro method for determination of pH, carbon dioxide tension, base excess and standard biocarbonate in capillary blood, Scand. J. Clin. Lab. Invest. 12:172, 1960.
42. Operator's Manual 113-S1, UM pH/Blood Gas System (Instrumentation Laboratory, Inc., Catalogue #79131, 1968).
43. Operator's Manual 213, pH Blood Gas Analyzer (Instrumentation Laboratory, Inc., Catalogue #79110, 1973).
44. Operator's Manual 513, pH/Blood Gas Analyzer and Acid-Base Calculator (Instrumentation Laboratory, Inc., Catalogue #79513, 1974).
45. Crampton Smith, A., and Hahn, C. E. W.: Electrodes for the measurement of oxygen and carbon dioxide tensions, Br. J. Anaesth. 41:731, 1969.
46. Lunn, J. N., and Mapleson, W. W.: The Severinghaus P_{CO_2} electrode: a theoretical and experimental assessment, Br. J. Anaesth. 35:666, 1963.
47. Adams, A. P., Morgan-Hughes, J. O., and Sykes, M. K.: pH and blood gas analysis, Anaesthesia 23:47, 1968.
48. Severinghaus, J. W., Stupfel, M., and Bradley, A. F.: Accuracy of blood pH and P_{CO_2} determinations, J. Appl. Physiol. 9:189, 1956.
49. Severinghaus, J. W.: Measurements of blood gases: P_{O_2} and P_{CO_2}, Ann. N.Y. Acad. Sci. 148:115, 1968.
50. Holmes, P. L., Green, H. E., and Lopez-Majano, V.: Evaluation of methods for calibration of O_2 and CO_2 electrodes, Am. J. Clin. Pathol. 54:566, 1970.
51. Linden, R. J., Ledsome, J. R., and Norman, J.: Simple methods for the determination of the concentrations of carbon dioxide and oxygen in blood, Br. J. Anaesth. 37:77, 1965.
52. Van Slyke, D. D., and Neill, J. M.: The determination of gases in blood and other solutions by vacuum extraction and manometric measurement, J. Biol. Chem. 61:523, 1924.
53. Sandroy, J., Jr., Dillon, R. T., and Van Slyke, D. D.: Studies of gas and electrolyte equilibria in blood, J. Biol. Chem. 105:597, 1934.
54. Peters, J. P., and Van Slyke, D. D.: *Quantitative Clinical Chemistry* (Baltimore: Williams & Wilkins Co., 1932) vol. II, p. 781.

55. Riley, R. L., Proemmel, D. D., and Franke, R. E.: A direct method of determination of oxygen and carbon dioxide in blood, J. Biol. Chem. 161:621, 1945.

56. Stow, R. W., Baer, R. F., and Randall, B. F.: Rapid measurement of the tension of carbon dioxide in blood, Arch. Phys. Med. Rehabil. p. 646, October 1957.

57. Severinghaus, J. W., and Bradley, A. F.: Electrodes for blood Po_2 and Pco_2 determinations, J. Appl. Physiol. 13:515, 1958.

58. Krebs, W. M., and Haddad, I. A.: The oxygen electrode in fermentation systems, Dev. Indust. Microbiol. 13:113, 1972.

59. Kreuzer, F., Watson, T. R., Jr., and Ball, J. M.: Comparative measurements with a new procedure for measuring the blood oxygen tension in vitro, J. Appl. Physiol. 12:65, 1958.

60. Heitmann, H., Buckles, R. G., and Laver, M. B.: Blood Po_2 measurements: Performance of microelectrodes, Respir. Physiol. 3:380, 1967.

61. Polgar, G., and Forster, R. E.: Measurement of oxygen tension in unstirred blood with a platinum electrode, J. Appl. Physiol. 15:706, 1960.

62. Sproule, B. J., et al.: An improved polarographic method for measuring oxygen tension in vitro, J. Appl. Physiol. 11:365, 1957.

63. Baumberger, J. P.: Determination of the oxygen dissociation curve of oxyhemoglobin by a new method, Am. J. Physiol. 123:10, 1938.

64. Berggren, S. M.: The oxygen deficit of arterial blood caused by nonventilating parts of the lung, Acta Physiol. Scand. 4:9(Suppl.11), 1942.

65. Clark, L. C., Jr.: Monitor and control of blood and tissue oxygen tensions, Trans. Am. Soc. Artif. Intern. Organs 2:41, 1956.

66. Bageant, R. A.: Oxygen analyzers, Respir. Care 21:5, 1976.

67. Willard, H. H., Merritt, L. L., and Dean, J. A.: Instrumental Methods of Analysis (New York: D. Van Nostrand Co., Inc., 1965).

68. Siggaard-Andersen, O., Norgaard-Pedersen, B., and Rem, J.: Hemoglobin pigments. Spectrophotometric determination of oxy-, carboxy-, met-, and sulfhemoglobin in capillary blood, Clin. Chim. Acta 42:85, 1972.

69. Malenfant, A. L., et al.: Spectrophotometric determination of hemoglobin concentration and percent oxyhemoglobin and carboxyhemoglobin saturation, Clin. Chem. 14:789, 1968.

70. Maas, A. H. J., Hamelink, M. L., and De Leeuw, R. J. M.: An evaluation of HbO_2, HbCO and Hb in blood with the Co-Oximeter IL 182, Clin. Chim. Acta 29:303, 1970.

71. Operator's Manual 182. Co-Oximeter (Instrumentation Laboratory, Inc., Catalogue #79182, 1975).

72. Nunn, J. F.: Nomograms for calculation of oxygen consumption and respiratory exchange ratio, Br. Med. J. 4:18, 1972.

73. Lavoisier, A. L.: Sur les altérations qui arrivent à l'air dans plusiers circonstances où se trouvent les hommes réunis en société, Mémoires de Médecine en Histoire de la Société de Médecine 5:569 (1782–1783, read in 1785).

74. Priestley, J.: The Discovery of Oxygen, Alembic Club Reprints (Chicago: The University of Chicago Press, 1906).

75. Bert, P.: Barometric Pressure: Researches in Experimental Physiology, transl. M. A. Hitchcock and F. A. Hitchcock (Columbus, Ohio: Longs College Book Co., 1943).

76. Cohen, P.: The metabolic function of oxygen and biochemical lesions of hypoxemia, Anesthesiology 37:148, 1972.
77. Warrell, D. A., *et al.:* Pattern of filling in the pulmonary capillary bed, J. Appl. Physiol. 32:346, 1972.
78. Caro, C. G.: Mechanics of the Pulmonary Circulation, in *Advances in Respiratory Physiology* (London: Arnold Publishing Ltd., 1966).
79. Halmaggi, D. F. J., *et al:* Pulmonary alveolar-vascular reflex, J. Appl. Physiol. 19:105, 1964.
80. Harvey, R. M., *et al.:* A reconsideration of the origins of pulmonary hypertension, Chest 59:82, 1971.
81. Hughes, J. M. B., *et al.:* Effect of lung volume on the distribution of pulmonary blood flow in man, Respir. Physiol. 4:58, 1968.
82. Fry, D. L.: Pulmonary mechanics: A unified analysis of the relationship between pressure, volume and gas flow in the lungs of normal and diseased human subjects, Am. J. Med. 29:672, 1960.
83. Macklin, C.: The pulmonary alveolar mucoid film and the pneumonocytes, Lancet 1:1099, 1954.
84. Pattle, R.: Surface Tension and the Lining of the Lung Alveoli, in Caro, C. (ed.): *Advances in Respiratory Physiology* (London: Arnold Publishing Ltd., 1966).
85. Bellingham, A. J., *et al.:* Regulatory mechanisms of haemoglobin oxygen affinity in acidosis and alkalosis, J. Clin. Invest. 50:700, 1971.
86. Benesch, R., *et al.:* Effect of organic phosphates from the human erythrocyte on the allosteric properties of hemoglobin, Biochem. Biophys. Res. Commun. 26:162, 1967.
87. Finch, C., and Lenfant, C.: Oxygen transport in man, N. Engl. J. Med. 286:407, 1972.
88. Bryan-Brown, C. W., *et al.:* Consumable oxygen: Availability of oxygen in relation to oxyhemoglobin dissociation, Crit. Care Med. 1:17, 1973.
89. Severinghaus, J. W.: Blood gas calculator, J. Appl. Physiol. 21:1108, 1966.
90. Brewer, G. J., and Eaton, J. W.: Erythrocyte metabolism: Interaction with oxygen transport, Science 171:1205, 1971.
91. Miller, D., and Lichtman, M.: Clinical Implications of Altered Affinity of Hemoglobin for Oxygen, in *Hematology for Internists* (Boston: Little, Brown & Co., 1971).
92. Metcalfe, J., *et al.:* Decreased affinity of blood for oxygen in patients with low-output heart failure, Circ. Res. 25:47, 1969.
93. Torrance, J., *et al.:* Intraerythrocytic adaptation to anemia, N. Engl. J. Med. 283:165, 1970.
94. Kreuzer, F.: Facilitated diffusion of oxygen and its possible significance; a review, Respir. Physiol. 9:1, 1970.
95. Laver, M. B.: A fable of our time: Oxygen transport, or does the emperor have new clothes? Anesthesiology 36:105, 1972.
96. Comroe, J. H., *et al.:* The unreliability of cyanosis in the recognition of arterial anoxemia, Am. J. Med. Sci. 214:1, 1947.
97. Ravin, M. B., *et al.:* Contribution and thebesian veins to the physiologic shunt in anaesthetized man, J. Appl. Physiol. 20:1148, 1965.
98. Riley, R. L., and Cournand, A.: Analysis of factors affecting partial pressures of oxygen and carbon dioxide in gas and blood of lungs: theory, J. Appl. Physiol. 4:77, 1951.

99. Riley, R. L., and Permutt, S.: Venous admixture component of the AaPO$_2$ gradient, J. Appl. Physiol. 35:430, 1973.
100. Biscoe, T. J.: Carotid body: Structure and function, Physiol. Rev. 51:437, 1971.
101. Woodbury, D. M.: Physiology of Body Fluids, in *Physiology and Bio-physics* (Philadelphia: W. B. Saunders Co., 1965).
102. Stern, L. I., *et al.:* Estimation of non-respiratory acid-base abnormalities, J. Appl. Physiol. 27:21, 1969.
103. Schwartz, W. B., *et al.:* The internal distribution of hydrogen ions with varying degrees of metabolic acidosis, J. Clin. Invest. 36:373, 1957.
104. Symposium. Current concepts of acid-base measurements. Ann. N.Y. Acad. Sci. 133:1, 1966.
105. Winters, R. W.: Terminology of acid-base disorders, Ann. Intern. Med. 63:873, 1965.
106. Bartels, H., *et al.:* Glossary on respiration and gas exchange, J. Appl. Physiol. 34:549, 1973.
107. Perkins, J. F., Jr.: Historical Development of Respiratory Physiology, in *The Handbook of Physiology, Respiration,* vol. 1 (Washington, D.C.: American Physiological Society, 1964).
108. Williams, H. M.: Ventilatory failure, Medicine 45:317, 1966.
109. West, J. B.: Causes of carbon dioxide retention in lung disease, N. Engl. J. Med. 284:1232, 1971.
110. Campbell, E. J. M., *et al.: The Respiratory Muscles, Mechanics and Neural Control* (London: Lloyd-Luke, 1970).
111. Otis, A.: The work of breathing, Physiol. Rev. 34:449, 1954.
112. McIlroy, M., *et al.:* The effect of added elastic and non-elastic resistances on the pattern of breathing in normal subjects, Clin. Sci. 15:337, 1956.
113. Von Euler, C., *et al.:* Control mechanisms determining rate and depth of respiratory movements, Respir. Physiol. 10:93, 1970.
114. Bartlett, R., *et al.:* Oxygen cost of breathing, J. Appl. Physiol. 12:413, 1958.
115. Peters, R.: The energy cost (work) of breathing, Ann. Thorac. Surg. 7:51, 1969.
116. Campbell, E., *et al.:* Simple methods of estimating oxygen consumption and efficiency of the muscles of breathing, J. Appl. Physiol. 11:303, 1957.
117. Eichenholz, A., *et al.:* Pattern of compensatory response to hypercapnia in patients with chronic obstructive pulmonary disease, J. Lab. Clin. Med. 68:265, 1966.
118. Elliott, R., and MacCorquodak, K. (eds.): *Elementary Statistics* (New York: Appleton-Century-Crofts, Inc., 1954).
119. Oldham, P. D.: *Measurement in Medicine: The Interpretation of Numerical Data* (London: English Universities Press, 1968).
120. Fleischer, W. R., and Gambiro, S. R.: *Blood pH, Pco$_2$, Po$_2$ and Oxygen Saturation* (4th ed.; Chicago: American Society of Clinical Pathology, Council on Clinical Chemistry, 1972).
121. Severinghaus, J. W.: Blood Gas Concentrations, in *The Handbook of Physiology, Respiration,* vol. II (Washington, D.C.: American Physiological Society, 1965).

122. Severinghaus, J. W.: Measurements of blood gases: P_{O_2} and P_{CO_2}, Ann. N.Y. Acad. Sci. 148:115, 1968.
123. Williams, R. J.: Standard human beings versus standard values, Science 126:453, 1957.
124. Elkinton, J. R.: Acid-base disorders and the clinician, Ann. Intern. Med. 63:893, 1965.
125. Asmussen, E., and Nielsen, M.: Physiologic deadspace and alveolar gas pressures at rest and during muscular exercise, Acta Physiol. Scand. 38: 1, 1956.
126. Jones, N. L., et al.: Physiological deadspace and alveolar-arterial gas pressure differences during exercise, Clin. Sci. 31:19, 1966.
127. Higgs, B. E., et al.: Changes in ventilation, gas exchange and circulation during exercise in normal subjects, Clin. Sci. 32:329, 1967.
128. Bergman, N. A.: Effect of varying respiratory wave forms on distribution of inspired gas during artificial ventilation, Am. Rev. Respir. Dis. 100: 518, 1969.
129. Hedenstierna, G., and McCarthy, G.: Mechanics of breathing, gas distribution, and functional residual capacity at different frequencies of respiration during spontaneous and artificial ventilation, Br. J. Anaesth. 47: 706, 1975.
130. Koch, G.: Alveolar ventilation, diffusing capacity and the A − P_{O_2} difference in the newborn infant, Respir. Physiol. 4:168, 1968.
131. Davies, C. T. M.: The oxygen-transporting system in relation to age, Clin. Sci. 42:1, 1972.
132. Muiesan, G., et al.: Respiratory function in the aged, Bull. Physiopathol. Respir. 7:973, 1971.
133. Kitamura, H., et al.: Postoperative hypoxemia: the contribution of age to the maldistribution of ventilation, Anesthesiology 36:244, 1972.
134. Jarboe, T. M., et al.: Ventilatory failure due to metabolic alkalosis, Chest 61:615, 1972.
135. Cohen, R., and Overfield, E.: The diffusion component of arterial hypoxemia, Am. Rev. Respir. Dis. 105:532, 1972.
136. Collier, C. R., et al.: Use of extracellular base excess in diagnosis of acid-base disorders: A conceptual approach, Chest 61:65, 1972.
137. Eriksen, H. C., and Sorensen, H. R.: Arterial injuries: Iatrogenic and noniatrogenic, Acta Chir. Scand. 135:133, 1969.
138. Mortensen, J. D.: Clinical sequelae from arterial needle puncture cannulation and incision, Circulation 35:1118, 1967.
139. Mathieu, A., et al.: Expanding aneurysm of the radial artery after frequent puncture, Anesthesiology 38:401, 1973.
140. Sackner, M. A., Avery, W. G., and Sokolowski, J.: Arterial puncture by nurses, Chest 59:97, 1971.
141. Barnes, R. W., et al.: Noninvasive assessment of altered limb hemodynamics, and complications of arterial catheterization, Radiology 107:505, 1973.
142. Kazamias, T. M., et al.: Blood pressure measurement with Doppler ultrasonic flowmeter, J. Appl. Physiol. 30:585, 1971.
143. Allen, E. V.: Thromboangiitis obliterans: Methods of diagnosis of chronic occlusive arterial lesions distal to the wrist with illustrative cases, Am. J. Med. Sci. 178:237, 1929.

144. Greenhow, D. E.: Incorrect performance of Allen's test—Ulnar artery flow erroneously presumed inadequate, Anesthesiology 37:356, 1974.

145. Richards, R. L.: *Peripheral Arterial Disease, A Physician's Approach* (Edinburgh and London: E. & S. Livingstone, 1970).

146. Ryan, J. F., *et al.:* Arterial dynamics of radial artery cannulation, Anesth. Analg. 52:1017, 1973.

147. Petty, T. L., Bigelow, B., and Levine, B. E.: The simplicity and safety of arterial puncture, J.A.M.A. 195:181, 1966.

148. Bageant, R. A.: Variations in arterial blood gas measurements due to sampling techniques, Respir. Care 20:565, 1975.

149. Kloster, F. E., Bristow, J. D., and Griswold, H. E.: Femoral artery occlusion following percutaneous catheterization, Am. Heart J. 79:175, 1970.

150. Barnes, R. W., *et al.:* Complications of brachial artery catheterization: Prospective evaluation with the Doppler ultrasonic velocity detector, Chest 66:363, 1974.

151. Barnes, R. W., *et al.:* Safety of brachial arterial catheters as monitors in the intensive care unit—prospective evaluation with the Doppler ultrasonic velocity detector, Anesthesiology 44:260, 1976.

152. Bjork, L., *et al.:* Local circulatory changes following brachial artery catheterization, Vasc. Dis. 2:283, 1965.

153. Katz, A. M., *et al.:* Gangrene of the hand and forearm: A complication of radial artery cannulation, Crit. Care Med. 2:270, 1974.

154. Downs, J. B., Chapman, R. L., and Hawkins, I. F.: Prolonged radial-artery catheterization, Arch. Surg. 108:671, 1974.

155. Barnes, R. W., *et al.:* Complications of percutaneous femoral arterial catheterization, prospective evaluation with the Doppler ultrasonic velocity detector, Am. J. Cardiol. 33:259, 1974.

156. Wyatt, R., Glaves, I., and Cooper, D. J.: Proximal skin necrosis after radial artery cannulation, Lancet 1:1135, 1974.

157. Bedford, R. F., and Wollman, H.: Complications of percutaneous radial-artery cannulation: An objective prospective study in man, Anesthesiology 38:228, 1973.

158. Dalton, B., and Laver, M. B.: Vasospasm with an indwelling radial artery cannula, Anesthesiology 34:194, 1971.

159. Hersey, F. B., and Calman, C. H.: *Atlas of Vascular Surgery* (St. Louis: C. V. Mosby Co., 1963).

160. Wigger, H. J., Bransilver, B. R., and Blanc, W. A.: Thromboses due to catheterization in infants and children, J. Pediatr. 76:1, 1970.

161. Johnson, R. W.: A complication of radial-artery cannulation, Anesthesiology 40:598, 1974.

162. Stamm, W. E., *et al.:* Indwelling arterial catheters as a source of nosocomial bacteremia—an outbreak caused by flavobacterium species, N. Engl. J. Med. 292:1099, 1975.

163. Davison, R., Shapiro, B. A., and Harrison, R. A.: Unpublished data.

164. Gardner, R. M., *et al.:* Percutaneous indwelling radial-artery catheters for monitoring cardiovascular function: Prospective study of the risk of thrombosis and infection, N. Engl. J. Med. 290:1227, 1974.

165. Walton, J. R., and Shapiro, B. A.: Unpublished data.

166. Bourke, D. L.: Errors in hematocrit determination, Anesthesiology 45:357, 1976.

167. Banister, A.: Comparison of arterial and arterialized capillary blood in infants with respiratory distress, Arch. Dis. Child. 44:726, 1969.
168. Dell, R. B., and Winters, R. W.: Capillary blood sampling for acid-base determinations — technique and validity, Radiometer, Copenhagen, #AS48.
169. Docrat, K., and Kenny, S.: The accuracy of capillary sampling for acid-base estimations, Br. J. Anaesth. 37:840, 1965.
170. Gandy, G., et al.: The validity of pH and PCO_2 measurements in capillary samples in sick and healthy newborn infants, Pediatrics 34:192, 1964.
171. Glasgow, J. F. T., Flynn, D. M., and Swyer, R. R.: A comparison of descending aortic and "arterialized" capillary blood in the sick newborn, Can. Med. Assoc. J. 106:660, 1972.
172. Jung, R. C., Balchum, O. J., and Massey, F. J.: The accuracy of venous and capillary blood for the prediction of arterial pH, PCO_2 and PO_2 measurements, Am. J. Clin. Pathol. 45:129, 1966.
173. Koch, G.: The validity of PO_2 measurement in capillary blood as a substitute for arterial PO_2, Scand. J. Clin. Lab. Invest. 21:10, 1968.
174. Koch, G., and Wendel, H.: Comparison of pH, carbon dioxide tension, standard bicarbonate and oxygen tension in capillary blood and in arterial blood during the neonatal period, Acta Paediatr. Scand. 56:10, 1967.
175. Laughlin, D. E., McDonald, J. S., and Bedell, G. N.: A microtechnique for measurement of PO_2 in "arterialized" earlobe blood, J. Lab. Clin. Med. 64:330, 1964.
176. Mountain, K. R., and Campbell, D. G.: Reliability of oxygen tension measurements on arterialized capillary blood in the newborn, Arch. Dis. Child. 45:134, 1970.
177. Siggaard-Andersen, O.: Acid-base and blood gas parameters — arterial or capillary blood? Scand. J. Clin. Lab. Invest. 21:289, 1968.
178. Galvis, A. G., Donahoo, J. S., and White, J. J.: An improved technique for prolonged arterial catheterization in infants and children, Crit. Care Med. 4:166, 1976.
179. Neal, W. A., et al.: Umbilical artery catheterization: Demonstration of arterial thrombosis by aortography, Pediatrics 50:6, 1972.
180. Tooley, W. H.: What is the risk of an umbilical artery catheter? Pediatrics 50:1, 1972.
181. Gupta, J. M., Roberton, N. R. C., and Wigglesworth, J. S.: Umbilical artery catheterization in the newborn, Arch. Dis. Child. 43:382, 1968.
182. Cochran, W. D., Davis H. T., and Smith, C. A.: Advantages and complications of umbilical artery catheterization in the newborn, Pediatrics 42:769, 1968.
183. Gambino, S. R., and Thiede, W. H.: Comparisons of pH in human arterial, venous and capillary blood, Am. J. Clin. Pathol. 32:298, 1959.
184. Phillips, B., and Peretz, D. I.: A comparison of central venous and arterial blood gas values in the critically ill, Ann. Intern. Med. 70:745, 1969.
185. Shapiro, H. M., et al.: Errors in sampling pulmonary artery blood with a Swan-Ganz catheter, Anesthesiology 40:291, 1974.
186. Evers, W., Racz, G. B., and Levy, A. A.: A comparative study of plastic (polypropylene) and glass syringes in blood gas analysis, Anesth. Analg. 50:92, 1972.
187. Scott, P. V., Horton, J. N., and Mapleson, W. W.: Leakage of oxygen from

blood and water samples stored in plastic and glass syringes, Br. Med. J. 3:512, 1971.

188. Winkler, J. B., *et al.:* Influence of syringe material on arterial blood gas determinations, Chest 66:518, 1974.

189. Rosenthal, T. B.: The effect of temperature on the pH of blood and plasma in vitro, J. Biol. Chem. 173:25, 1948.

190. Gambino, S. R.: Heparinized vacuum tubes for determination of plasma pH, plasma CO_2 content, and blood oxygen saturation, Am. J. Clin. Pathol. 32:285, 1959.

191. Report of the ad hoc committee on acid-base terminology of the New York Academy of Sciences conference: Current concepts of acid-base measurement, Ann. N.Y. Acad. Sci. 133:251, 1966.

192. Yoshimura, H.: Effects of anticoagulants on the pH of the blood, J. Biochem. (Tokyo) 22:297, 1935.

193. Kelman, G. R., and Nunn, J. F.: Nomograms for correction of blood Po_2, Pco_2, pH and base excess for time and temperature, J. Appl. Physiol. 21: 1484, 1966.

194. Simkins, T.: Quality control: Undefined and underused, J. Cardiovasc. Pulm. Tech. 2:19, 1974.

195. Cissik, J. H., and Salustro, J.: Quality control of arterial blood gas analysis, J. Cardiovasc. Pulm. Tech. 3:25, 1975.

196. Serrette, C.: A system of quality control of blood gas analysis, Respir. Ther. 5:41, 1975.

197. Komjathy, Z. L., *et al.:* Stability and precision of a new ampuled quality control system for pH and blood gas measurements, Clin. Chem. 22: 1399, 1976.

198. Oliver, W. R., and Golden, S.: Quality control of pH and Pco_2 blood gas analyses. Presented at the 2d annual meeting of the N.S.C.P.T., May, 1969.

199. Chalmers, C., Bird, B. D., and Whitwam, J. G.: Evaluation of a new thin film tonometer, Br. J. Anaesth. 46:253, 1974.

200. Ravin, M. B., and Briscoe, W. A.: Blood gas transfer, hemolysis, and diffusing capacity in a bubble tonometer, J. Appl. Physiol. 19:784, 1964.

201. Flenley, D. C., Millar, J. S., and Rees, H. A.: Accuracy of oxygen and carbon dioxide electrodes, Br. Med. J. 2:349, 1967.

202. Nunn, J. F.: Oxygen tension temperature factor, Anesthesiology 27:204, 1966.

203. Burton, C. W.: Measurement of inspired and expired oxygen and carbon dioxide, Br. J. Anaesth. 41:723, 1969.

204. Elliott, S. E., *et al.:* A modified oxygen gauge for the rapid measurement of Po_2 in respiratory gases, J. Appl. Physiol. 21:1672, 1966.

205. Dripps, R. D., Eckenhoff, J. E., and Vandam, L. D.: *Introduction to Anesthesia* (4th ed.; Philadelphia: W. B. Saunders Co., 1972).

206. Wylie, W. D., and Churchill-Davidson, H. C.: *A Practice of Anaesthesia* (2d ed.; Chicago: Year Book Medical Publishers, Inc., 1970).

207. Riley, R. L., *et al.:* "Ideal" alveolar air and the analysis of ventilation-perfusion relationships in the lungs, J. Appl. Physiol. 1:825, 1949.

208. King, T. K. C., and Briscoe, W. A.: Rise in arterial oxygen saturation breathing 24% oxygen in chronic lung disease, J. Appl. Physiol. 32:776, 1972.

209. Davidson, F. F., *et al.*: The components of the alveolar-arteriolar oxygen tension difference in normal subjects and in patients with pneumonia and obstructive lung disease, Am. J. Med. 52:754, 1972.

210. Weil, J. V., and Zwillich, C. W.: Assessment of ventilatory response to hypoxia: Methods and interpretation, Chest 70:124, 1976.

211. King, T., and Briscoe, W.: Abnormalities of blood gas exchange in COPD, Postgrad. Med. 54:101, 1973.

212. Robin, E. D.: Abnormalities of acid-base regulation in chronic pulmonary disease, with special reference to hypercapnia and extracellular alkalosis, N. Engl. J. Med. 268:917, 1963.

213. Clark, J. M., and Lambertsen, C. J.: Pulmonary oxygen toxicity: A review, Pharmacol. Rev. 23:37, 1971.

214. Severinghaus, J. W., *et al.*: Alveolar deadspace as an index of distribution of blood flow in pulmonary capillaries, J. Appl. Physiol. 10:335, 1957.

215. Hey, E. N., *et al.*: Effects of various respiratory stimuli on the depth and frequency of breathing in man, Respir. Physiol. 1:193, 1966.

216. Deal, C. W., *et al.*: Veno-arterial shunting in experimental pulmonary embolism, J. Surg. Res. 10:579, 1970.

217. Wilson, J. E., *et al.*: Hypoxemia in pulmonary embolism, a clinical study, J. Clin. Invest. 50:481, 1971.

218. Fisher, S. R., *et al.*: Comparative changes in ventilatory deadspace following micro and massive pulmonary emboli, J. Surg. Res. 29:195, 1976.

219. Duranceau, A., *et al.*: Ventilatory deadspace in diagnosis of acute pulmonary embolism, Surg. Forum 25:229, 1974.

220. Freeman, J., and Nunn, J. F.: Ventilation-perfusion relationships after haemorrhage, Clin. Sci. 24:135, 1963.

221. Johansson, H., and Lofstrom, J. B.: Effects on breathing mechanics and gas exchange of different inspiratory gas flow patterns during anesthesia, Acta Anaesthesiol. Scand. 19:8, 1975.

222. Bergman, N. A.: Effect of varying respiratory waveforms on distribution of inspired gas during artificial ventilation, Am. Rev. Respir. Dis. 100:518, 1969.

223. Otis, A. B., *et al.*: Mechanical factors in distribution of pulmonary ventilation, J. Appl. Physiol. 8:427, 1956.

224. Morris, R. C.: Renal tubular acidosis, N. Engl. J. Med. 281:1405, 1969.

225. Weil, M. H., *et al.*: Experimental and clinical studies on lactate and pyruvate as indications of the severity of acute circulatory failure (shock), Circulation 41:989, 1970.

226. Jarboe, T. M., *et al.*: Ventilatory failure due to metabolic alkalosis, Chest 61:615, 1972.

227. DeRubertis, F. R., *et al.* Complications of diuretic therapy: Severe alkalosis and syndrome resembling inappropriate secretion of anti-diuretic hormone, Metabolism 19:709, 1970.

228. Kassirer, J. P., *et al.*: The critical role of chloride in the correction of hypokalemic alkalosis in man, Am. J. Med. 38:172, 1965.

229. Schwartz, W. B., *et al.*: Role of anions in metabolic alkalosis and potassium deficiency, N. Engl. J. Med. 279:630, 1968.

230. Hamilton, W. K.: Atelectasis, pneumothorax and aspiration as postoperative complications [review], Anesthesiology 22:708, 1961.

231. Sellery, C. R.: A review of the causes of postoperative hypoxia, Can. Anaesth. Soc. J. 15:142, 1968.

232. Petty, T., et al.: The adult respiratory distress syndrome, Chest 60:233, 1971.

233. Moore, F.: Post Traumatic Pulmonary Insufficiency (Philadelphia: W. B. Saunders Co., 1969).

234. McFadden, E. R., Jr., et al.: Arterial blood gas tension in asthma, N. Engl. J. Med. 278:1027, 1968.

235. Loeb, H. S., et al.: Effects of low-flow oxygen on the hemodynamics and left ventricular function in patients with uncomplicated acute myocardial infarction, Chest 60:352, 1971.

236. Robin, E. D., et al.: Pulmonary edema, N. Engl. J. Med. 288: 239, 1973.

237. Miller, A., et al.: Acute, reversible respiratory acidosis in cardiogenic pulmonary edema, J.A.M.A. 216:1315, 1971.

238. Tattersfield, A. E., et al.: Relationship between hemodynamic and respiratory function in patients with myocardial infarction and left ventricular failure, Clin. Sci. 42:751, 1972.

239. Duncalf, D., et al.: Ventilatory requirements after open-heart operations, Anesth. Analg. 49:518, 1970.

240. Thung, N., et al.: The cost of respiratory effort in postoperative cardiac patients, Circulation 28:552, 1963.

241. Addington, W. W., et al.: Cystic fibrosis of the pancreas—a comparison of the pulmonary manifestations in children and young adults, Chest 59: 306, 1971.

242. Gaensler, E. A., et al.: Pulmonary function in pregnancy, Am. Rev. Tuberc. 67:779, 1953.

243. Lucius, H., et al.: Respiratory functions, buffer system and electrolyte concentrations of blood during human pregnancy, Respir. Physiol. 9:311, 1970.

244. Boutros, A., et al.: Management of carbon monoxide poisoning in the absence of hyperbaric oxygenation chamber, Crit. Care Med. 4:144, 1976.

245. Downs, J. B.: Personal communication.

246. Harrison, R. A., et al.: Unpublished data.

247. Fick, A.: Ueber die Messung des Blutquantums. in dem Herzventrikeln. Sitzungsb. der phys.-med. Ges. zu Wurzburg: 1870, 36.

248. Forster, R. E.: Exchange of gases between alveolar air and pulmonary capillary blood: Pulmonary diffusing capacity, Physiol. Rev. 37:391, 1959.

249. Prys-Roberts, C., Kelman, G. R., and Greenbaum, R.: The influence of circulatory factors on arterial oxygenation during anesthesia in man, Anaesthesia 22:257, 1967.

250. Otis, A. B.: Quantitative Relationships in Steady State Gas Exchange, in The Handbook of Physiology, Respiration, vol. 1 (Washington, D. C.: American Physiological Society, 1964).

251. Cournand, A., et al.: Measurements of cardiac output in men using the technique of catheterization of the right auricle or ventricle, J. Clin. Invest. 24:106, 1945.

252. Pontoppidan, H., et al.: Medical progress: Acute respiratory failure in the adult, N. Engl. J. Med. 287:743, 1972.

253. Harrison, R. A., *et al.:* Reassessment of the assumed A-V oxygen content difference in the shunt calculation, Anesth. Analg. 54:198, 1975.
254. Forrester, J. S., *et al.:* Filling pressure in the right and left sides of the heart in acute myocardial infarction, N. Engl. J. Med. 285:190, 1971.
255. Rosenbaum, R. W., *et al.:* The importance of pulmonary artery pressure monitoring, Surg. Gynecol. Obstet. 136:261, 1973.
256. Ellertson, D. G., *et al.:* Pulmonary artery monitoring in critically ill surgical patients, Am. J. Surg. 128:791, 1974.
257. Stevens, P. M., *et al.:* The value of flow directed catheter in cardiorespiratory failure, Am. Rev. Respir. Dis. 107:1111, 1973.
258. Unger, K. M., *et al.:* Detection of left ventricular failure in patients with adult respiratory distress syndrome, Chest 67:8, 1975.
259. Sutter, P. M., *et al.:* Optimal end-expiratory airway pressure in patients with acute pulmonary failure, N. Engl. J. Med. 292:284, 1975.
260. Lee, J., *et al.:* Central venous oxygen saturation in shock, Anesthesiology 36:472, 1972.
261. Swan, H. J. C., *et al.:* Catheterization of the heart in man with use of a flow-limited balloon-tipped catheter, N. Engl. J. Med. 283:447, 1970.
262. Zierler, K. L.: Circulation Times and the Theory of Indicator Dilution Methods for Determining Blood Flow and Volume, in *Handbook of Physiology, Circulation,* vol. 1 (Washington, D.C.: American Physiological Society, 1962).
263. Harrison, R. A., *et al.:* Unpublished data.
264. Woods, M., *et al.:* Practical considerations for the use of a pulmonary artery thermister catheter, Surgery 79:469, 1976.
265. Branthwatte, M. A., *et al.:* Measurement of cardiac output by thermal dilution in man, J. Appl. Physiol. 24:434, 1968.
266. Wessel, H. U., *et al.:* Limitations of thermal dilution curves for cardiac output determinations, J. Appl. Physiol. 30:643, 1971.

Index